HEALTHFUL EATING WITHOUT CONFUSION

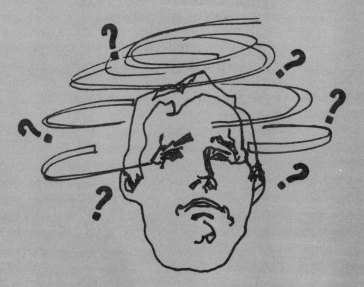

By
PAUL C. BRAGG, N.D., Ph.D.
Life Extension Specialist

with

PATRICIA BRAGG Ph. D.

Published by

Health Science

Box 477, Desert Hot Springs, California 92240, U.S.A.

HEALTHFUL
EATING
WITHOUT CONFUSION

By
PAUL C. BRAGG, N.D., Ph.D.
Life Extension Specialist

with

PATRICIA BRAGG Ph. D.

Published in the United States, Australia and England by
HEALTH SCIENCE - Box 477, Desert Hot Springs, California 92240 U.S.A.

Library of Congress Catalog Card Number: 71-152392

ISBN: 0-87790-024-8

Printed in the United States of America

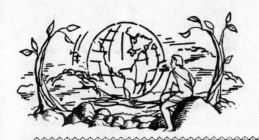

CONTENTS

RONALD O'NEAL

CONTENTS

RONALD O'NEAL

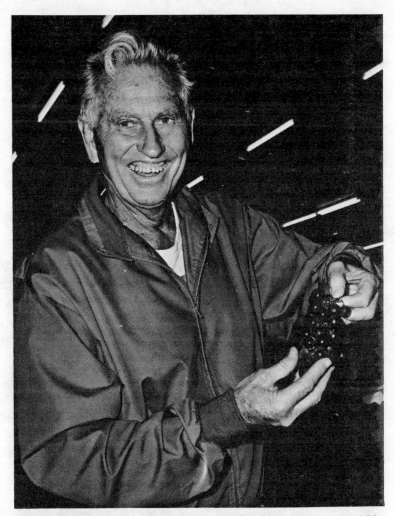

Paul C. Bragg lives on live, living foods. Grapes are one of his favorite fruits, as they are a source of high energy.

UNCOMPLICATE YOUR LIVING

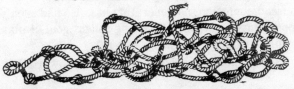

Living is a continual lesson in problem solving, but the trick is to know where to start. No excuses — start your Health Program Today.

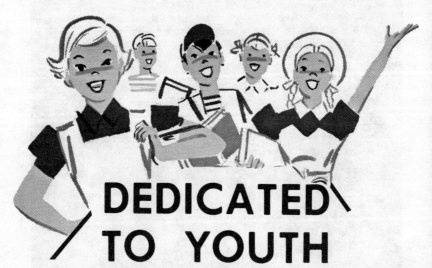

DEDICATED
TO YOUTH

Probably no generation has been born into such widespread confusion as today's youth! And paramount in that confusion is the basic problem of healthful nutrition — upon which the solution of all other problems ultimately depends. A healthy mind in a healthy body is the prime essential in coping with any and all other difficulties — from sex to world peace.

Here is where I can help. As the world's oldest practicing biochemist and nutritionist, I have had the time and opportunity to evaluate carefully the numerous and varied dietetic theories that have been foisted on the public during this twentieth century.

This book brings you the benefit of my experience. Here is an authenticated guide to lead you out of the labyrinth of nutritional confusion . . . to the diet best suited to the proper and healthful functioning of your own body chemistry.

It is dedicated to Youth of All Ages — for you are never too young or too old to start on the Road to Health!

But the sooner the better. This book, therefore, is especially dedicated to the Youth of Today — for, ironically, in spite of the widespread confusion, no generation has also had such widespread opportunity to achieve that long-sought goal of mankind — an alert mind in an ageless body.

Follow the guidance of this book . . . and start toward that goal today!

Paul C. Bragg

HEALTHFUL
EATING
WITHOUT CONFUSION

NUTRITIONAL CONFUSION

My lecture and nutritional research takes me all over the world. When people learn that I am a biochemist and nutritionist, they invariably say something like this:

"I've been wanting to change my diet to achieve better health. But the more I investigate this subject, the more confused I become. None of you nutritionists seem to agree on anything! How do you expect a person like me to find a way to better health through nutrition, when all I find is utter confusion among the so-called experts?"

Day after day, hundreds of letters come to my office in Burbank, California with the same sort of frustrated questions. These individuals — of all ages — are sincerely interested in proper nutrition but completely confused by the conflicting advice from real and pseudo-nutritional "experts".

And I will have to agree with these intelligent health-seekers. The whole field of nutrition is riddled with confusion. It is a hodgepodge of contradictions. It is like a jig-saw puzzle that cannot be solved. No matter what one diet expert has to say, there are a hundred others who will say he is absolutely wrong.

How can anyone determine which diet is right for him? In my long career in this field, I have found certain infallible guideposts that point the way. Let me share these with you.

FOOD IS THE MAGIC HEALER

Five hundred years before the birth of Christ, **Hippocrates — the father of the natural healing sciences — said** . . .

"Food will be your medicine, and medicine will be your food."

Hippocrates further stated,

"Strength, growth, nourishment result from the right food."

These statements are equally true today. We know that the only real cures come from food.

As an example, let's take scurvy, the disease that kills thousands around the world every year. It can definitely be cured by

1

massive doses of vitality Vitamin C. Beri-beri is another dreaded deficiency disease, for which massive doses of Vitamin B-Complex can effect a cure. The same goes for many forms of anemia, which can be cured only by an adequate amount of iron and copper. Malnutrition, which is a syndrome of many nutritional deficiencies, can be cured by a perfectly balanced diet.

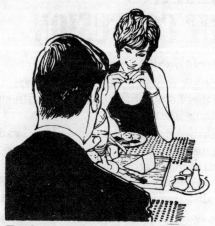

Food can make or break you. You can dig your grave with your knife, fork and spoon.

I could go on and on telling of the importance of nutrition in ridding the body of diseases. No drugs can make such claims. Food is the magic healer. Keep constantly in mind that . . .

"Food will be your medicine, and medicine will be your food."

Food can make or break you!
What you eat today will be walking and talking tomorrow!

AMERICANS ARE OVERFED — BUT POORLY NOURISHED!

Travel the world over, and in no country will you find the abundance of food that the United States produces. Go into the supermarkets of any city or town in the U.S.A. and you will find the shelves loaded with every imaginable kind of food.

No country in the world can boast of having as many restaurants as we have. You can purchase finger-licking fried chicken in barrels, pizza pies, hot cakes, hot dogs, hamburgers, delicatessen foods, steaks and chops, Italian food, Greek food, Chinese food, Polish food, Kosher food, Japanese food, French food, English food, Mexican food, Hungarian food . . . you name the food and you can purchase it.

Yet with all this great array of food, we are poorly nourished. And the hidden hungers of the overfed are as much cause for concern as the food deficiencies of the underfed.

Did you notice the sunbathers at the beaches this summer? There may have been a lot of wellformed youngsters — but there were also a lot of skinny and fat ones, too. And most of the older sunbathers were examples of what these young people would become if they should — as is all too likely — continue on the usual American diet. Most of the adults were in poor physical condition — many of them flabby, fat, overstuffed and paunchy.

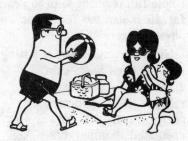

Americans tend to be over-weight!

Being overfed can be even more dangerous than being un-derfed, unless one is really starved. Just as there is malnourishment among the poor, there is also malnourishment among the well-to-do. In both cases, important nutrients are missing in the daily diet. Too much rich food — such as fatty meats, dairy products, eggs, sugary and salty foods — are just as dangerous to good health as too little.

HIDDEN HUNGERS OF THE OVERFED

Just who are these people who are overfed yet poorly nourished? They include:

- Any child or adult who is 20 or more pounds overweight.
- Any child or adult who is moderately anemic because of low hemoglobin, the blood pigment containing iron and copper which carries oxygen to the body cells.
- Any adult male whose cholesterol level is above normal.
- Any child or adult who is rundown and tired all the time.
- Any person who is nervous.
- Any person who has trouble with his eyes, teeth, bones.

These are among the more obvious symptoms that reveal the hazards of vitamin, mineral and enzyme deficiencies. There are many more.

If a man can convince me that I do not think or act right, gladly will I change, for I search after truth. But he is harmed who abideth on still in his ignorance.
— *Marcus Aurelius, Roman Emperor*

LOOK AT "UNCLE BILL"

To give you an illustration, let's look at "Uncle Bill". Most of us have one — an overfed, undernourished relative or friend. Uncle Bill is about 45 to 55 years old, and 25 or more pounds too fat. He is just too heavy and awkward to get any pleasure out of physical exercise.

His main enjoyment is sitting before the TV eating and drinking. He likes beer, cola drinks and coffee. He relishes salty popcorn, candy bars, hot dogs, cremated hamburgers, greasy fried chicken, slices of pizza pie, cookies, cakes, doughnuts, salty nuts and other empty calorie, foodless food.

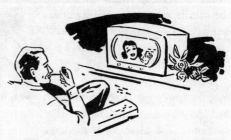

Sitting before TV eating, drinking and smoking is a deadly habit!

His diet is filled with too many empty calories and loaded with saturated fats that crowd cholesterol into his bloodstream. His beverages are filled with refined white sugar which throws his metabolism off balance.

To top it all, his wife loads the table at each meal with rich foods. She feeds him a big breakfast under the illusion that "it will give him strength". She makes rich pancakes, piled high with butter and dripping with rich, sugary syrup, accompanied by big slices of bacon, ham or pork sausage. She serves him fried eggs, hot cereals covered with refined white sugar and rich cream or milk. She prides herself on her delicious, rich and creamy desserts.

DIET OF DEATH

This kind of eating has been Uncle Bill's diet most of his life. His wife is feeding him the same kind of food that his mother did when he was growing up. He has survived up to now because of a naturally strong constitution, and because during his youth and early married years he was physically active and thus used up and eliminated a good deal of the excess sugar and cholesterol.

Now fat and fiftyish, Uncle Bill unthinkingly continues his diet of death — boasting proudly that he has **"a cast-iron stomach."**

But what is really happening inside Uncle Bill's body? Even working overtime, his already overstrained vital organs cannot cope with the excess salt, sugar and cholesterol. Mineral deposits are hardening the once elastic walls of his arteries and

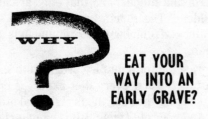
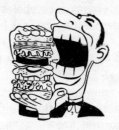

WHY EAT YOUR WAY INTO AN EARLY GRAVE?

other blood vessels, which are also being narrowed by fatty deposits which could easily trap a blood clot. If this should occur in a vessel of the heart or the brain, it could spell death for poor Uncle Bill.

In a heart attack, the coronary arteries are affected. With a stroke, the blood vessel damage is in the brain.

A heart attack can be a frightening experience and it starts many people thinking about the role of diet in avoiding another one. This is what happens with Uncle Bill. His doctor has told him that he has a deadly disease, arteriosclerosis, and that the condition will probably continue and even accelerate, unless he changes his diet.

CONFUSION INSTEAD OF SOLUTION

Now Uncle Bill is cured, and he promises himself that he will find the correct way to eat to avoid another heart attack. He has been advised to buy some books on nutrition, so he goes to a

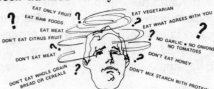

bookstore and asks to see the section on good diet. After a careful examination of the books, he purchases four.

Americans searching for healthful eating habits find confusion among diet experts.

To Uncle Bill's amazement, he discovers that each book has a different theory on correct diet. One tells of the glories of being a strict vegetarian, asserting that a complete vegetarian diet will prevent a heart attack. The next book, however, says just the opposite — that meat, eggs and dairy products are necessary for healthful living. The third book is all for an entirely raw food diet. It states that cooked food is unfit to eat, that milk and milk products produce cholesterol and mucus, and that eggs are also dangerous cholesterol builders. The fourth book sets forth the superiority of a fruitarian diet — declaring that fruit and nuts are the only perfect food for man.

Here is poor Uncle Bill grasping for a dietary program to save him from another heart attack — and every diet expert is contradicting the other, each insisting that only he is right and other authorities are all wrong. And poor old Uncle Bill is caught right in the middle of this confusion about correct nutrition.

MY EARLY EXPERIENCE

In writing this book, I am not producing "**just another diet book**" to add further confusion to a very confused subject. Instead, I am going to help you see that there is a way to design a correct diet for yourself with all the confusion completely eliminated.

To begin with, my life was saved by the science of nutrition. At the age of 16, I had a terminal case of T.B. By the grace of God, I was led to Dr. August Rollier in Leysin, Switzerland, a man who was a hundred years ahead of his time in the science of nutrition. From a boy dying with a vicious disease — for whom not one doctor or sanatarium in America could hold out any hope of recovery — I became a healthy young man!

Dr. Rollier put me on a diet of whole foods — raw fruit and vegetables, properly cooked vegetables, whole natural cheese (made from milk from healthy animals who had no medication and no food sprayed with poisonous insecticides). I was fed eggs from fertile hens, meat — especially lamb — three times a week, bread made from freshly ground wholegrain rye, raw nuts, seeds, beans, plenty of garlic, apple cider, grape juice, dates, sun dried figs and apricots.

In less than two years I was not merely an arrested case of T.B. — I was completely cured!

The Doctor of the future will give no medicine but will interest his patents in the care of the human frame, in diet and in the cause and prevention of disease.
— Thomas A. Edison

SEVENTY YEARS LATER

Ever since my recovery I have had a painless, tireless, ageless body. I have been an outstanding athlete in many sports. And today, as a great-grandfather, I am still an athlete — at the age when most men of my calendar years are half dead, senile, feeble old people with one foot in the grave.

I still jog, swim miles at a time, climb some of the world's highest mountains, play fast tennis, practice progressive weight training with barbells and dumbells. I write several books a year, and have a lecture schedule that takes me around the globe. Plus, I continue my intense research on nutrition and life extension.

I am a product of well balanced nutrition. As far as I know, I am the oldest full time practicing nutritionist alive.

I still have all my own teeth, and a scalp full of healthy hair. My blood pressure is 124/78, and I have a strong, steady pulse of 64. My 20/20 vision is as keen as an eagle's, and my hearing as sharp as an alert animal's.

Let me state again that, from a terminal case of T.B. in my teens, I have attained this vigorous great-grandfatherhood through proper nutrition.

Furthermore, I number my health students in the tens of thousands from all over the world. I have received many thousands of unsolicited testimonials telling me what my books on diet and health have accomplished for many once helpless sick people. Many state that after reading my books and following my advice they have been "reborn".

Therefore, I believe that with my many years of scientific background in nutrition, I can help you to help yourself!

Every man is the builder of a temple called his body . . . We are all sculptors and painters, and our material is our own flesh, blood and bones. Any nobleness begins at once to refine a man's features, any meanness or sensuality to imbrute them.
— Henry David Thoreau

To my mind the greatest mistake a person can make is to remain ignorant when he is surrounded, every day of his life, by the knowledge he needs to grow and be healthy and successful. It's all there. We need only to observe, read, learn . . . and apply.
— Paul C. Bragg

NOTED DENTIST RESEARCHES PRIMITIVE DIETS
AROUND THE WORLD

Dr. Weston Price, a dentist from Cleveland, Ohio, author of **"Nutrition and Physical Degeneration"**, goes down as one of the 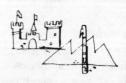 world's greatest nutritionists. Dr. Price traveled throughout the world studying the eating habits of primitive peoples. He also studied their teeth, dental arches and bone structure, their freedom from disease, their energy, vitality and endurance, and their length of life.

To his amazement, he found healthy, vigorous, long lived people whose eating habits varied widely. There were those who ate a mixed diet of meat, eggs, fish, poultry, whole grains, fruit and vegetables, 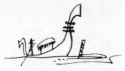 dairy products, beans, nuts, seeds and sea vegetables. He found others, just as healthy, who were strict vegetarians and never touched any food coming from an animal.

He studied the healthy Laplanders, who lived on reindeer meat in a bitterly cold climate. He found healthy tribes living in the steaming jungles of Africa on a diet of

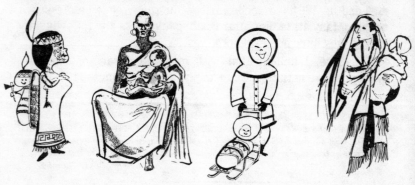

Primitive diets of natural, unprocessed foods produce healthy, happy people!

raw milk and blood. He found the beautiful, strong Polynesians of the South Sea Islands thriving on a diet of poi, made from the root of the taro plant, raw and cooked fish, and an abundance of fresh tropical plants.

Dr. Price's worldwide research revealed that there are people living long, healthy lives in all kinds of climates, eating the natural foods of their environment — foods close to nature.

MY OWN RESEARCH ON PRIMITIVE NUTRITION

My own researches among primitive peoples living completely away from civilization parallels that of Dr. Price. I found all types of people living in all sorts of climates, who were disease free, vigorous at advanced ages, with powerful bodies, perfect teeth, eyes, ears and vital organs.

Did they all eat the same diet? Absolutely not! There were healthy meat eaters, healthy vegetarians, and healthy mixed eaters.

In neither Dr. Price's research nor mine did we find different primitive peoples following the same diet. Their eating habits were as varied as the climates in which they lived.

PRIMITIVE PEOPLES HEALTH
THE SECRET — NATURAL FOODS!

Yes, the diets of these primitive peoples showed wide variety — but they all had an important nutritional factor in common. They ate the foods which were natural to their particular environment.

None of them ate any refined white sugar. They never ate anything made in a factory, which is perverted with all kinds of chemical additives and artificial processing.

They did not eat packaged foods, ice cream, candy — no hot dogs, smoked meats, preserved meats or delicatessen foods. They did not use tobacco in any form. They drank no alcohol, coffee, tea, chocolate or cola drinks.

All the food of these primitive peoples was organically grown, in natures' way. It was free from artificial commercial fertilizers, from poisonous sprays and pesticides. They ate no canned or frozen foods. Except for the raw milk drinkers, very few of those studied used dairy products. They were free from mucus, and their cholesterol count was low.

THE DEVASTATION OF CIVILIZATION

These primitive peoples, whom Dr. Price and I studied, were uncontaminated by civilization. Living as nature intended them to live, they were free from the miseries and diseases that plague civilized man.

We are always hearing what civilization is doing for us — but we seldom, if ever, hear what it is doing to us to destroy our health and our life.

Whole races have been wiped out and are being wiped out after introduction of the dead, devitalized diet called "civilized". In my lifetime, I have witnessed the almost utter destruction of the noble Hawaiian race from this cause.

When I first came to these Islands in 1912, there were many Hawaiians still living on their native foods . . . including an abundance of sea-food, the basic "poi" from the taro root, and a large variety of tropical fruit such as avocado, passion fruit, bananas and many more. In the districts where these people lived, I examined their teeth, dental arches and their whole physical bodies. They were wonderful specimens of healthy human beings, in every respect.

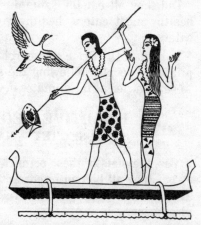

Primitive Hawaiians were healthy!

Take their teeth, for example. Among the Hawaiians who maintained their native diet, dental cavities or caries were only 2 per cent.

In contrast, the Hawaiians who had adopted the white man's diet of refined white flour products, refined white sugar, white rice, processed meats (such as hot dogs and luncheon meats), commercial dry cereals, canned goods and other dead-foods of civilization, showed 60 to 80 per cent tooth decay. Many were suffering from degenerative diseases.

10

On each subsequent visit that I make to these lovely Islands of the Pacific — where I am now writing this book — I find the noble Hawaiian race dying out more and more rapidly. It is being wiped out by malnutrition and physical degeneration, the results of our devastating civilization.

The same is true in many of the South Sea Islands, which I visit in my continuing research on nutrition and health. Many island groups realize that their people are doomed, melting away with degenerative diseases. Their one overwhelming desire is that their race shall not die out. They know that something serious and terrible has happened since they have been encroached upon by the civilization and the deadly refined foods and dead-foods of the white man.

Surely, our civilization is on trial both at home and abroad!

THE WHITE MAN IS COMMITTING SLOW SUICIDE

The effects of our Western civilization's diet of death on other races is more rapid and therefore more apparent than what we are doing to ourselves. But the white man is eating his way out of existence. He is committing slow suicide on a racial scale.

This has been going on for a long time in ignorant bliss. Today, however, the very confusion about nutrition is a symptom that we are, at least, aware that something is wrong.

That this awakening is taking place is borne out by the many "Uncle Bill" letters which I receive — as often from the distressed wife as from "Uncle Bill" himself.

Even more encouraging is the interest in nutrition among "Uncle Bill's" sons and daughters, nieces and nephews. I am receiving more and more inquiries from the parents of young families and even from teenagers. More and more college students and young working adults are among the audiences at my lectures.

Their questions are intelligent. They have become aware of the importance of proper nutrition, and are seeking their way out of the maze of confusion on this subject. Health Food Stores throughout the country report a growing number of young people among their customers.

It is this sort of thing that has stimulated me to write this book. There is still time to turn the tide from self-destructive eating habits that could engulf the race and send it into oblivion through slow suicide.

There is still time for civilized man to rejuvenate himself and take a new lease on life by proper eating habits. He may not be able to return to the natural foods of his ancestors — but he can take advantage of natural, organically grown foods in his own environment.

ANCIENT MAN WAS HEALTHIER THAN WE ARE

Ancient man was a much healthier animal than modern man, according to Dr. Robert D. McCracken, University of California (UCLA) anthropologist. Although people often think that 20th century man lives longer than 17th or 18th century man, McCracken points out that longevity figures are a statistical anomaly.

What we have done by our conquest of infectious diseases, better housing, modern sanitation, rapid and widespread distribution of fresh fruits and vegetables the year around, and other hygienic factors is to save the lives of infants and young people. This has increased the number of old people — and therefore extended the life span averages.

McCracken said that the first coronary attack was not medically described until early in this century. A famous Boston cardiologist, Dr. Paul Dudley White, once said that he never heard of a coronary while he was in medical school.

Modern man's devitalized diet is responsible for his pervasive ill health, according to McCracken, who stated that man "is basically a meat and fruit eating animal." He said that refined white sugar is to a large extent to blame for some forms of diabetes, heart disease, stroke, schizophrenia, alcoholism and even possibly some kinds of cancer.

"Living under conditions of modern life, it is important to bear in mind that the perparation and refinement of food products either entirely eliminates or in part destroys the vital elements in the original materials." — **U.S. Dept. of Agriculture**

"Now learn what and how great benefits a temperate diet will bring with it.
In the first place, you enjoy good health.
— **Horace, 65-8 B.C.**

NATURAL SUGARS ARE HEALTHFUL

Refined white sugar was not used among the healthy primitive peoples whose eating habits were researched by both Dr. Price and me. They used no synthetic manufactured sugars such as sucaryl or saccharin. In fact, they did not even use raw or brown sugar.

Some of them used honey in moderation. But the great majority got their sugar from their general natural diet of organically grown fruits and vegetables. That is why these people had such excellent teeth, and were free from the dreaded gum disease pyorrhea, as well as from other degenerative diseases of civilization.

Poor nutrition, refined sugars and their many products, soft drinks, sweets, etc., are causing epidemic tooth decay and gum diseases among Americans.

THE IMPORTANCE OF INSULIN BALANCE

Professor McCracken noted that sugar is the ultimate energy provided by foods, but that the rate at which it is absorbed by the body determines whether or not it causes metabolic abnormalities to develop. The faster the rate of absorption, the greater the number of abnormalities.

Habitual consumption of refined white sugar and foods containing it in a readily absorbed form upsets the delicate balance between too low and too high sugar levels. And that is just what modern man does — eats too much rapidly absorbed refined white sugar and its products.

McCracken reported that when sugar enters the bloodstream, insulin is secreted by the pancreas to facilitate its passage through cell membranes of the tissues, where it is used as fuel.

Normal secretion of insulin by the pancreas is two thimbles full daily. If too much readily absorbed sugar enters the bloodstream, however, an excess of insulin may be secreted. Ironically, this condition causes the blood sugar level to fall.

Walk in the path of duty, do good to your brethren, and work no evil towards them.
— **Chao Hun K'ung**

HYPOGLYCEMIA — THE GREAT MASQUERADER!

The essential point is that if the insulin itself is not controlled, the blood sugar falls to abnormally low levels. This condition is known as hypoglycemia.

Researchers are beginning to call hypoglycemia **"the great masquerader"** because, like syphilis, it presents so many apparently unrelated symptoms.

These symptoms are triggered by the brain, which is the organ most sensitive to low blood sugar caused by the attempt of the pancreas to restore the balance. The brain is a very sensitive biochemical organ, in which fully 25% of the adult body's metabolic activity takes place. When the blood sugar gets too low, as it does when large amounts of insulin are secreted to control rapidly absorbed refined white sugar, the brain begins to malfunction. It freaks out.

REFINED WHITE SUGAR IS POISON

Refined white sugar is not only absolutely worthless as an item of nourishment in the diet, but it is also extremely dangerous to life and health in the great quantities in which most people consume it in desserts, beverages, candy, cake, ice cream and the thousands of other commercial products in which it is used.

As noted by McCracken, the great indictment against refined white sugar is its high solubility in the body. It rushes through the stomach wall without being digested, stimulates excess secretion of insulin by the pancreas, and causes metabolic imbalances which permit bacteria, viruses and deadly germs to get a firmer foothold.

Sugar is definitely fattening. It has been found dangerous for heart cases, as it disorganizes the calcium-phosphorous balance in the blood. In large quantities, as previously noted, it causes the blood sugar level to drop too low, which could produce mental and other serious troubles.

To clinch his argument that refined white sugar rather than fats is to blame for many of modern man's degenerative diseases, anthropologist McCracken cited certain primitive tribes who consume many more saturated fats than Western man, but who never touch refined white sugar or its products. These people, he reported, have very low blood cholesterol levels, and very

14

few of the diseases to which we in the West fall victim. He calls refined white sugar "the worst thing man can eat."

The same opinion was expressed by a dentist to whom I was talking a few days ago. He stated that more dentures (full uppers and lowers) are now being made and placed in the mouths of thousands of children and adults, whose teeth have deteriorated chiefly because of a diet containing a quantity of refined white sugar.

An even higher price to pay for tastebud thrills is diabetes, whose victims face the threat of blindness and other serious impairments. Not to mention heart troubles, skin diseases and a host of other ailments that result from eating this white poison.

AMERICANS ARE ON A SWEET-TOOTH BINGE

According to a recent AP food situation report, the per capita consumption of refined white sugar in the United States has increased by many pounds over previous years. Today it is about 105 pounds per year, twice as much as in 1870. The use of refined white sugar in the manufacture of foods and beverages is reported to have climbed to an all-time high.

And it is precisely during the past century — during which the per capita consumption of refined white sugar has doubled — that degenerative diseases have assumed such devastating importance in the morbidity and mortality statistics.

Americans today are on a refined white sugar sweet-tooth binge. **We are truly a nation of "sugarholics".** And what a price we are paying!

Flesh is dumb . . . you can put anything in your mouth and swallow it. It takes brains to manage what goes into your body!

> **Read the labels on all manufactured, bottled and canned goods . . . and if it says "SUGAR" drop it as you would poison!**

A NATURAL DIET IS SALT-FREE!

Nutritional research among primitive peoples reveals that very, very few of them use salt. Fortunately, many tribes live where salt is not available — miles from salt mines or the sea. Others, even when salt is available, have acquired no taste for it. Their diet of fresh, organically grown fruit and vegetables —

free from artificial fertilizers and chemicals — provides them with an ample supply of natural organic minerals and vitamins.

Even primitive tribes who live in hot, steaming jungles find no need for salt in their diet.

For flavor, these peoples use natural herbs in cooking. Such dishes are far more delicious, as well as nutritious, than those in which salt is used. Natural herbs bring out the natural flavors of foods. Salt kills the original taste.

My own studies, and those of other authorities, show that these people who live on a natural, salt-free diet are free from arteriosclerosis, kidney diseases, dropsy, high blood pressure, skin diseases, obesity and baldness — all ailments of Western man in which salt is a deadly factor.

SALT — THE KILLER!

Inorganic sodium chloride, or common table salt, is indigestible by the human body or that of any other animal. Only plants can transform inorganic minerals, including sodium, into an organic form suitable for human and animal nourishment. The so-called "craving for salt" is due to a lack of natural organic minerals in the diet.

Although salt has been used in the human diet for thousands of years, this is not because the body needs it. Salt is an acquired, artificial taste, which developed because salt was the first and is still the most extensively used food preservative discovered by man. Even in this modern age of refrigeration and other mechanical marvels, man continues to use salt to lengthen the life of his food — and shorten his own life!

Because salt is indigestible, it must either be eliminated from the human body or stored in water soluble form. You can readily see what an overload salt puts upon the kidneys, and how body tissues — and finally vital organs — become waterlogged from the storage of non-eliminated salt.

Salt can also cause incrustations in the arteries, veins and capillaries, narrowing and hardening the walls of these blood vessels. To force the blood through these damaged vessels, the heart must increase its pressure. The Japanese, who have the highest blood pressure of any people in the world, are also the world's heaviest consumers of salt.

STAGES OF
ARTERY HARDENING

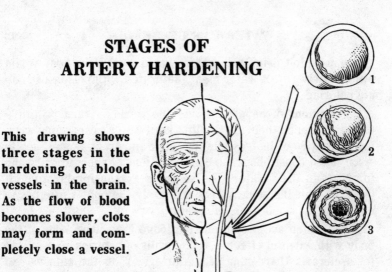

This drawing shows three stages in the hardening of blood vessels in the brain. As the flow of blood becomes slower, clots may form and completely close a vessel.

The annual consumption of salt in the United States now amounts to more than 100 pounds per capita, and is constantly increasing. So is the incidence of high blood pressure, dropsy, edema, kidney and liver ailments, arteriosclerosis, congestive heart failure, and other miseries of the human body caused by the eating of salt and salty foods.

Salt is an insidious killer! It paralyzes the 260 taste buds in the mouth, creating an unnatural craving or addiction by deadening certain of the body's warning signals.

If you are a salt-eater, you are an addict. Withdrawal from this inorganic poison, however, does not produce the drastic symptoms such as drug withdrawal. You may be nervous and a bit uncomfortable at first, while your body rids itself of this unwelcome burden and your taste buds recover from the salt-induced paralysis and return to normal.

In about six weeks, you will not only feel more alive and vigorous — but you will also savor the varied, delicate, true flavors of the foods you eat. Be sure your diet includes plenty of fresh fruits and vegetables, which will supply your body with all the organic sodium it needs, as well as pure distilled water.

17

WATER CAN BE DEADLY

You wouldn't drink salt water, would you? Your body would immediately reject water highly saturated with poisonous sodium chloride.

Yet millions of people all over the world — even primitive tribes — quench their thirst with "hard water" containing varying quantities of indigestible inorganic minerals. Some "health spas" even boast about the concentrations of specific inorganic minerals in their water. The so-called "cleansing laxative effect" of drinking such waters is merely the body's attempt to eliminate these inorganic minerals.

Those which are not eliminated lodge in various parts of the body with harmful effect — in the walls of arteries, causing arteriosclerosis (hardening of the arteries); in the kidneys and gall bladder, producing painful stones; in the movable joints, stiffening these into an arthritic condition; on the bones, forming hurtful spurs.

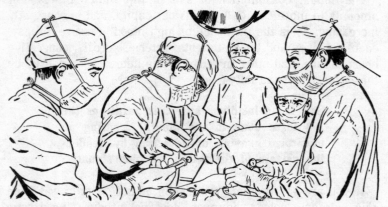

There are nearly eight thousand hospitals in the U.S.A. Surgery goes on around the clock. Many people go into surgery to have painful spurs removed, also bladder stones, kidney stones and gall stones. Will you be next?

My book, **"The Shocking Truth About Water"**, discusses these dangerous effects in detail, as well as the additional hazards of the inorganic chemicals so extensively used to "purify" urban drinking water.

SEVEN TYPES OF JOINTS
WHERE TROUBLE BEGINS

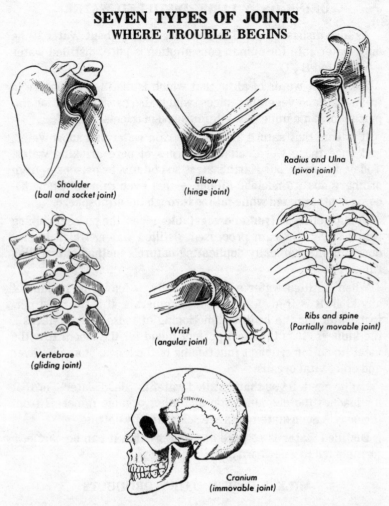

Shoulder
(ball and socket joint)

Elbow
(hinge joint)

Radius and Ulna
(pivot joint)

Vertebrae
(gliding joint)

Wrist
(angular joint)

Ribs and spine
(Partially movable joint)

Cranium
(immovable joint)

These are the seven types of joints in your body that have movement. Between each of these moveable joints there is a clear amber fluid called synovial fluid which acts as a lubricant to keep the joints moving easily. When inorganic minerals from drinking water and toxic acid crystals replace this synovial fluid we have stiffness, pain and misery.

It is my conviction, after more than sixty years of nutritional research, that the key factor in most human ills is the drinking of impure water — and that includes naturally "hard" water.

DRINK ONLY PURE, DISTILLED WATER

As also discussed in **"The Shocking Truth About Water,"** the only water safe for human consumption is pure, distilled water — undiluted H_2O.

The purest water of all is that which is distilled by nature in fresh fruit and vegetable juices, which also carry in solution important organic minerals, vitamins and nutrients.

It is true that nature also distills rain water and snow water, and once these were reliable sources of pure drinking water. Today, however, our Earth's air is so polluted by poisons — from ordinary dust to nuclear fallout — that even rain and snow become contaminated while falling through the atmosphere.

Outside of fresh fruit and vegetable juices, the purest drinking water today is steam processed distilled water, which is produced by mechanically duplicating nature's method of distilling rain.

When distilled water enters the body, it leaves no residue of any kind. It is free of all inorganic minerals. It is the most perfect water for the healthy functioning of those great "sieves", the kidneys. It is the most perfect liquid for the blood. It is the ideal liquid for efficient functioning of the lungs, stomach, liver and other vital organs.

Let no one tell you that distilled water is "dead water", or that it "leaches the calcium, iron and other organic minerals from the body". Such statements are scientifically untrue.

Distilled water is so pure and healthy that it can be part of a formula fed to a newborn baby.

MILK & OTHER DAIRY PRODUCTS

Pure milk, especially mother's milk, is indeed "nature's most perfect food" — for babies. But no animal on the face of the earth — except man — drinks fluid milk after it is weaned. In fact, in most countries throughout the world very little fluid milk is consumed by adults.

In America, however, milk is big business. Diet "experts" of the dairy industry tell the public about the wonders of pasteurized milk, exhorting everyone to drink a quart of milk a day for calcium to make strong bones and teeth.

These "experts" neglect to add that milk is a factor in making children grow tall, and that there is strong scientific evidence that very tall people are less healthy and shorter lived than the average. They suffer from diseases of the blood vessels in the legs, have a greater tendency to high blood pressure and foot and back troubles.

Also omitted is the fact that adults, having attained their normal bone growth, will assimilate only the amount of calcium necessary to their body chemistry. The residue of excess calcium can cause difficulties.

In my long experience as a nutritionist, I have found that too much milk causes heavy mucus conditions in the sinuses, throat, lungs and bowels. There are other adverse conditions which arise from drinking pasteurized and even raw milk after infancy.

Today's milk, due to the artificial practices of agriculture and the dairy industry, is not the wonderful old-fashioned raw milk of years ago. Cows are fed on material grown with chemical fertilizer and heavily saturated with pesticides. Most dairy cows never roam a green meadow or get sunshine. They spend their lives in cement barns, where milk is produced on an assembly line basis. This confinement makes for sick cows, to which various antibiotic injections are given.

Cheese made from the milk of these sick cows is heavily salted. Additives are put into commercial cottage cheese and yogurt for uniform eye and taste appeal. One group of scientists stated recently that commercial yogurt may be the cause of cataract, an eye disease in which the lens becomes opaque, producing partial or total blindness.

The most widespread blindness, however, is the fact that most Americans "eat with their eyes", demanding uniformity in the appearance of their foods. Only additives and chemicals, many of which are harmful to health, can accomplish this uniformity. Commercial ice cream is a chemical feast — don't eat it!

Always bear in mind that milk and all dairy products have a high cholesterol content. My suggestion is to go light on or discontinue pasteurized milk and its products, including buttermilk, salted butter, cheese, cottage cheese and yogurt.

Health consists with Temperance alone."
— **Pope**

DON'T EAT FRIED FOODS

Animal fat is saturated fat, also high in cholesterol. Ancient man, as primitive man today, converted much of this natural body fuel into physical energy. But modern man is a sedentary creature, who utilizes a comparatively small amount of cholesterol. As previously noted, the residue is deposited along the walls of the arterial and other blood vessels, causing dangerous clogging and clots.

CLOGGED PIPES

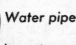

Water pipe

Artery

An artery with heavy internal deposit can be compared to scale that forms on the inside of a water pipe. An artery in this condition causes increase in blood pressure and may cause a heart attack or stroke.

For this reason more and more people are learning to use unsaturated fats such as safflower oil, soybean oil, and so on, because these fats are more easily assimilated into the body chemistry.

However, regardless of what kind of fat you use, the high temperatures required for frying — especially French-frying — destroy any food value the original fat might have had, and probably replace it with dangerous elements. In fact, heating fat over and over again for cooking use may be a possible cause of cancer.

Americans are a nation of stomach sufferers — chiefly because Americans live in haste and frying is the quickest way to

---

"To preserve health is a moral and religious duty, for health is the basis for all social virtues. We can no longer be useful when not well."
— Dr. Samuel Johnson, Father of Dictionaries

God sends the food, man by refining and processing foods destroys its nutritional value. Eat only God's natural foods.—Patricia Bragg

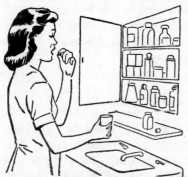

prepare food. Consider the number of hamburger stands all through this country, where cremated hamburgers are prepared on greasy grills and served with deep fat French-fried potatoes. There is no more indigestible combination!

If you don't believe me, listen to the predominating commercials on radio and TV, peddling this and that for relief of acid indigestion, sour stomach, gas bloat, heartburn, belching and a host of other stomach problems.

We are a nation of pill takers. Every 24 hours between 30 and 35 tons of aspirin alone is consumed.

DON'T EAT LEFTOVERS

Just as reheating of fat destroys food values, so double cooking of any foods is harmful. Every time you cook a food over again, you lose many of its natural nutrients.

Warmed over and recooked food means eating empty calories!

Many people think they are saving money by serving leftovers. They may be saving money, but they are surely looking for trouble nutritionally. In the Bragg household we throw away cooked food that has been previously served.

I have known of people who make a pot of soup with potatoes, rice and barley and keep reheating it, meal after meal, until it is finished. Little do they realize that they are serving their families bacterial soup. Cooked starches such as potato, rice and barley make a perfect culture for all kinds of deadly germs. As a result, tens of thousands of people suffer from severe ptomaine, and many die from eating food that is actually in a state of decay.

Why take chances with your health and life by eating leftover foods? Simply because leftover food is refrigerated does not save it from contamination.

23

Please do not be penny wise and health foolish! Remember, reheated foods are dead foods! In building a health diet for yourself, see how much live food you can put on the menu.

DANGEROUS NON-ALCOHOLIC BEVERAGES

Tea, coffee, cola drinks, soft drinks and chocolate drinks are all dangerous to your health. None of these has any live enzymes, vital nutrients, vitamins or organic minerals. So why put this "trash" into your wonderful body chemistry? It can do you no good — and it can really do your body a lot of harm!

Any kind of coffee, including the decaffinated kind, is a poison and an over-stimulant to your hardworking heart. It contains dangerous tars which foul up the liver, and uric acid which is a factor in stiffening your movable joints and hardening your arteries.

Tea is also a no-good beverage. It contains caffeine, tannic acid and theine, all of which are heavy toxic poisons that damage your wonderful body!

Cola and soft drinks are carbonated — and carbonated water works a hardship on your kidneys, bladder and other vital organs. These drinks are heavily sweetened with refined white sugar or its derivatives, plus the additional hazards of artificial coloring and flavoring.

Chocolate and chocolate beverages really give the liver a beating when it tries to cope with the many toxic materials they contain, chief among these is thiabromine, a toxin which destroys nerve cells. (Healthful desserts — you substitute carob which tastes just like chocolate — but contains only good nutrients.)

ALCOHOL IS A HEALTH WRECKER AND A KILLER!

The most damaging substance for your liver is alcohol. Every social and hard drinker of alcohol whom I knew fifty years ago in clubs and organizations is dead! Most of them died of cirrhosis of the liver, a degenerative disease which literally turns the liver into stone.

During my long life, I have seen many brilliant and intelligent men and women destroy themselves with alcohol. I have seen

24

wonderful homes broken up, and have known of terrible crimes committed while under the influence of this deadly poison.

Alcohol turns people into fools and life into a tragedy!

People tell me that their doctors have advised them to have a drink or two of alcohol to relax after a hard day at the office. I do not believe in this theory. Recent research has proven that it is a fallacy to regard alcohol as a relaxant, or that it is beneficial as a daily drink for older persons because it expands the arteries and stimulates circulation. I do admit that alcohol opens up the arteries temporarily, but the after-effect is harmful.

Alcohol is a thief that steals the important B-Complex Vitamins from the body. This seriously damages the central nervous system. As you have no doubt seen, an alcoholic is a trembling, nervous wreck. And there are 20 million chronic alcoholics in America today.

Drunken drivers are responsible for half the automobile accidents that take a huge toll in lives and permanent injuries. A person under the influence of alcohol loses all sense of intelligent reasoning as well as muscular coordination.

I am constantly being asked about wine and beer. People have read or have been told that one or both of these beverages are beneficial to health.

I have but one answer in regard to wine,
beer or any other alcoholic beverage:

Alcohol of any kind, no matter how small the dose, damages the liver, kidneys and bladder, and the tissues of the brain! Don't be confused about wine and beer. They are poisons. Keep them out of your body!

Admittedly, some people seem to get along all right with a small amount of alcohol every day, but they would certainly get along better without it.

The use of alcohol in any form indicates a deficiency in nutrients. The artificial stimulation of alcohol is only a substitute for nutritional deficiencies.

In my long practice as a Naturopathic doctor, I have helped chronic alcoholics to eliminate the alcohol habit completely and regain natural energy and vitality through a health program, which includes proper natural nutrition, vigorous exercise, deep breathing, and the use of natural food supplements especially the B-Complex Vitamins.

DON'T USE DRUGS INDISCRIMINATELY

Often people who come to me for nutritional advice will tell me of a certain medicinal drug which they "must keep on taking, regardless of diet."

My answer is, **"Oh ye of little faith! You do not have enough faith to believe that a program of proper nutrition will dispense with the drug."**

Consider high blood pressure, for example. As a Naturopathetic doctor, I have had a number of people come to me with very high blood pressure for which they were taking a special drug.

I immediately put them on a salt-free diet, with no dairy products, no meat, no eggs — a strict diet of only freshly steamed vegetables, fruit, seeds and nuts, with two 24-hour periods of fasting every week. And the elevated blood pressure came tumbling down!

At best, a drug is merely a crutch. People are always looking for something for nothing! They break the great laws of nature, get sick — and then expect a powerful drug to work like magic and get them well.

It is quite true that a drug may alleviate one disease — but it may produce another. We hear of "wonder drugs" such as cortisone, antibiotics, sulfa drugs, and so on . . . then sooner or later we hear of the dangerous side effects which these drugs produce.

Remember that a healthy body, completely nourished, withstands disease. No drug can cure any ailment. Only nature cures!

Find and follow the natural food diet best suited to your own body chemistry — and empty your medicine chest of pain killers, milk of magnesia, sleeping pills, antihistamines, tranquilizers, pep pills, fizzing bromides, bicarbonate of soda, aspirin, nose sprays, benezedrine, mineral oil, strong cathartics and other laxatives, and "nerve pills".

These "crutches" are part of a chain reaction, beginning with poor nutrition. Overfed but poorly nourished, the human body suffers from lack of natural nutrients . . . seeks to compensate for these deficiencies first with stimulants . . . then with medical drugs . . . and ultimately, in too many cases, with "hard drugs", the rapidly self-destructive narcotics and hallucigenics.

Reverse the process before it is too late! The symptoms which you attempt to relieve with drugs are warning signs from your sick body . . . nature's "S.O.S.".

Answer this call for help — not by palliatives — but by getting at the root cause.

Begin at the beginning. Feed your body with the nutrients it needs, and it will respond·amazingly. The human body is self-healing and self-repairing. But it must work with the material you supply — the food you put into your mouth. Give your body proper nutrition, and it will give you radiant health.

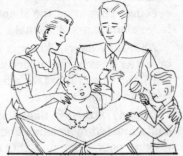

If this child were to live on a 100% Health Program it would have a Long Life and enjoy a Painless, Tireless and Ageless Body.

NEVER USE ALUMINUM COOKING WARE

Proper nutrition involves not only the correct selection of foods, but also their proper preparation. And even when you cook your food correctly, it may be spoiled by a chemical reaction with the wrong kind of cooking utensils.

Such is the case with aluminum ware, and also with the recently introduced Teflon ware.

When aluminum ware first came on the market many years ago it was — and still is — widely promoted for its convenience in use because of its light weight, and for its low cost.

I remember reading a book at that time by Dr. Betts, a dentist, who pointed out that aluminum is a soft metal and that, when used in cooking, some of it will dissolve into the hot water and combine with minerals in the food, often resulting in harmful contamination.

Not long ago I read of a tragic incident, similar to other instances of which I have read and heard.

In preparing a big fund-raising dinner, members of an organization used large aluminum pots for cooking some of the food the night before. The items were steamed string beans, chickens and rhubarb. When these were done, the volunteer cooks went home, leaving the food in the aluminum pots overnight.

The following morning other volunteers arrived to make

rhubarb pies for dessert at the big dinner scheduled for that evening. They used the rhubarb cooked and left overnight in a large aluminum pot, to make luscious looking, thick pies.

What they did not know is that, to begin with, rhubarb should be eaten in extreme moderation because of its oxalic acid content. And when this oxalic acid combines with aluminum, you are really in serious trouble.

Tragedy attended that dinner. The beans and chicken were contaminated by cooking and remaining almost 24 hours in aluminum pots . . . and the rhubarb was poisonous. Although stomach pumps were used in an attempt to get this poisoned food from the stomachs of the victims, twenty of the diners died of ptomaine poisoning and many others hovered at death's door for days.

Throw away every aluminum utensil you have in your kitchen. Immediately replace these with stainless steel, heavy enamelware or Pyrex.

I cannot recommend the new Teflon ware, although it has the advantage of enabling you to cook without grease. However, in time or after getting a hard blow, the treated surface may become opened or broken and a very toxic substance will then come in contact with your food. This toxin can cause severe digestive troubles.

Products such as Teflon are being developed as a result of the growing public awareness of the importance of proper nutrition. "Greaseless frying" has a definite commercial appeal. But, as noted, you should not use grease in any kind of utensil and you should not subject foods to high frying temperatures, with or without grease. New products which offer panaceas in the field of nutrition merely contribute to the growing confusion.

PROMOTERS OF NUTRITIONAL CONFUSION

By far the greatest contributors to nutritional confusion today are the big commercial food interests. Since they reap billions of dollars from the American people every year, they can well afford the millions they spend in advertising — in newspapers and magazines, on radio and TV — extolling the "nutritional" values of their devitalized, dead-food, supermarket products.

A large bread company, for example, claims that its refined

white flour bread, which is further adulterated by preservatives, "builds the body in 27 different ways" — when the truth of the matter is that if you fed this bread to a dog, he'd die in 15 days.

The refined sugar interests tell the public that refined white sugar is the most nourishing sweetener man can use — when the fact is that this empty-calorie, denatured sugar unbalances the body metabolism with often serious results.

The salt industry states that salt is a necessity in proper nutrition, and that iodized salt prevents goiter — when this inorganic mineral in reality acts as a poison in the human body.

To support these false claims, the powerful commercial food industries have subsidized an army of "dieticians" and "nutritionists" to brainwash the public.

These pseudo or "orthodox" nutritionists and dieticians have themselves been brainwashed in university and college courses in nutrition, which are dominated by commercial food producers.

BIASED COURSES IN NUTRITION

Nutrition is one of our youngest sciences. It has been only in the last few years that universities and colleges have offered courses in this subject.

As might be expected, the giant commercial food industry has dominated these courses. These commercial food interests are highly organized. They can see to it that the textbooks of courses in nutrition are keyed to their products.

These textbooks tell the students of nutrition to beware of the "food-faddist". They ridicule organically grown foods and claim that there is no harm in the use of chemical fertilizers and pesticides.

The mass produced, devitalized dead-foods distributed through the supermarkets of our nation are described as wonderful inventions of food science.

FALSE NUTRITIONAL PROPAGANDISTS

These mis-statements are parrotted by the graduates of these commercially controlled nutrition courses. They will tell you that Americans are the best fed people in the world, that modern processing has made our diet more wholesome and nutritious.

The pseudo or orthodox nutritionists and dieticians spread their false propaganda about the nutritional value of "junk" foods through every medium of communication, from TV to the public schools — "PTA" meetings, etc.

In commercials, lectures and conferences they will say that the human body can tolerate DDT and other poisonous sprays on food, that none of the poisonous food additives will harm you. In fact, they claim, such practices improve the quality of the food you eat.

Natural food nutritionists are labeled by these supermarket propagandists as "health nuts" and "food quacks". They invariably warn you to avoid Health Food Stores, "because health foods are more expensive and not as good as regular supermarket food."

They will tell you that refined white flour bread is better than whole-grain bread because it has been enriched with (synthetic) vitamins, that refined white sugar is an energy food, and that salt is an important item in nutrition.

> **Don't let these so-called nutrition "experts" confuse you! You know they are working in the interest of the big commercial food processors — and not for your health!**

YOUNG MOTHERS, BEWARE!

A favorite medium for these commercial dieticians and nutritionists is women's magazines. If you look through such magazines carefully, you will frequently find that articles on nutrition have an obvious tie-in with advertisers.

Among the most harmful of such articles are those telling young mothers all about the "splendid nutrition" found in commercial baby foods.

Don't you believe a word of it. Practically all commercial baby foods contain heavy concentrations of salt, refined white sugar, starch and monosodium glutinate. All these items are totally unfit for a baby to eat! Research has proved that they are dangerous to the baby's health.

If your food is debitalized, the important elements of nourishment have been removed, or if its value has been diminished by wrong cooking processes — you can then starve to death on a full stomach.

DON'T POISON YOUR BABY

A child's life is precious. Any woman who takes on the great responsibility of being a mother should purchase fresh fruit and vegetables and prepare them properly to feed her baby. It is worth every bit of the time and trouble required.

By teaching your child at an early age to enjoy fresh fruit and vegetables — first raw, then correctly cooked — you are giving your baby the best possible life insurance. You are starting him sturdily on the road to health and happiness.

Of course, it is so much easier to open a can or bottle of commercial baby food. It saves so much time and trouble. I have seen young mothers on trains and planes spooning this commercial mixture into babies' mouths. To me, it is a crime against a helpless baby to feed him that "junk".

I have seen mothers feed their children baby food that contained not only salt, refined white sugar, monosodium glutinate (MSG), but also such strong chemicals as benzoate of soda and sulfur dioxide. How can you build strong, healthy bodies with strong, unhealthy chemicals?

But mothers are feeding chemicalized foods to their babies every day. They have been brainwashed into believing that these are wholesome baby food.

Don't let the commercial dieticians confuse you. Commercial foods are not good baby food.

As for commercial baby cereals — not only are these devitalized and completely useless as food for any living thing, but no cereal of any kind should be fed to an infant. A child should not be given starch coming from a grain — even a whole grain cereal — until he is two years old. Prior to that age, children do not have the digestive juices to handle cereal food.

Up to age two, feed your child plenty of freshly steamed vegetables and fresh fruit (you can puree them in your blender) and freshly squeezed juices — orange, grapefruit, etc. Then, after two years old, start him on whole-grain cereal.

There are no more important ingredients of a properly constituted diet than fruits and vegetables, for the contain vitamins of every class, recognized and unrecognized.
— Sir Robert McCarrison

THE COMMERCIAL CEREAL HOAX

For fifty years I have been telling the world that there is practically no nourishment in commercial cereals. It took a recent Congressional investigation to prove that I was right. "The breakfast of champions" was revealed to be nothing but empty calories and empty promises!

The nutritional nonsense foisted upon the mothers of this country by the manufacturers of both dry and cooked commercial cereals is an insult to the intelligence. Before the cereal leaves the factory it has been murdered and is just a corpse of the grains, most of which is saturated with deadly refined white sugar. Eating the boxes in which the cereal comes would give more nutrition than eating the cereal.

These commercial cereals, both dry and cooked, have been processed to have an indefinite shelf life. They are so dead that bugs will not touch them — but the sad fact is that humans eat the stuff!

Powerful financially and with a powerful lobby in Washington, the commercial cereal manufacturers felt that no government agency could prevent them from telling any fairy story about their dead cereals that they wanted to.

Now that they have been called to task, they will change their pitch. But that will not necessarily change their product. Public memory is short lived, and people have become passive about being brainwashed by advertising.

The only factor that can force the commercial cereal companies and others of the giant food industry to improve the nutritional quality of their products is an aroused public resistance — a "protest march" away from the supermarket shelves, a widespread refusal to purchase the dead, devitalized foods that are sapping the strength of Western civilization.

THE PROGRESSIVE DECLINE OF MODERN CIVILIZATION

As long as civilized man continues to eat refined white sugar, and refined, bleached, degerminated, demineralized, devitamized and de-nutritionized white flour and its deadly products, salt and salty foods, white rice, chemicalized hot dogs and luncheon meats, hydrogenated foods, foods with chemical additives such as monosodium glutinate (MSG) and the many other varieties of dead-foods, there will be a decline of health and physical fitness.

That the rate of degeneration is progressively accelerating constitutes cause for great alarm.

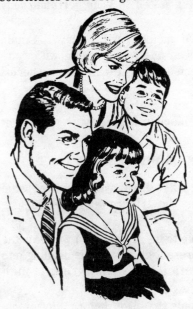

LIFE'S GREATEST TREASURE IS RADIANT HEALTH

"There is no substitute for Health. Those who possess it are richer than kings."

That is the reason I do not want you to be confused about nutrition. **We natural food nutritionists agree that the dead-foods must be eliminated from your diet.**

NATURAL NUTRITIONISTS AGREE ON BASICS

People often ask me why we natural food nutritionists do not agree 100% with one another.

I tell them that we do agree on the important basic aspects of nutrition:

1. Not to eat dead-foods, refined foods, processed foods and sprayed foods.

2. To eat natural foods which supply the body with essential nourishment, including organic minerals, vitamins and nutrients.

Just how to accomplish that second basic precept is where we find the variation in points of view. As I have said, nutrition is

33

one of our youngest sciences, and it will take time to make it an exact science. Today there is a shortage of efficiently and correctly trained nutritionists and biochemists.

So, to a certain extent, you will have to become your own nutritionist in selecting the diet best suited to your personal body chemistry.

To help guide you in this vital choice, I will review the main natural food diets that have been advocated, along with comments based upon my own experience and research over a period of some sixty years.

First, however, let us take up Precept No. 1, on which all natural food nutritionists and biochemists agree — i.e., what not to eat.

ELIMINATE DEAD-FOODS FROM YOUR DIET

"Tell me what you eat, and I will tell you what you are," said Jean Anthelme Brillat-Savarin, the 18th century French gastronome.

His aphorism is especially true today. The person who eats the dead, devitalized foods of our present civilization is heading into many complex nutritional deficiencies and terminal malnutrition.

Today we have more sick people than ever before, more mentally disturbed people, more crime, more young people addicted to a deadly drug habit. All this can be laid directly to the wretched nutrition to which modern man is subjected.

As my lectures and research work take me all over the world, I have the opportunity to meet and confer with the world's great biochemists and nutritionists. Speaking at many conventions of the National Health Federation, I again have the opportunity to hear and speak with many qualified nutritionists.

As noted, I have found that — although we may differ on the exact natural food diet to follow — we are all in basic agreement on the elimination from the diet of all devitalized, dead-foods.

THE "NO-NO" LIST — WHAT NOT TO EAT

Without fear of successful contradiction, I would state that most qualified nutritionists and biochemists agree that the following foods and beverages contribute absolutely nothing to the health and well-being of a human, and could be harmful.

"NO-NO"
FOODS NOT TO EAT:

A. General

1. Foods grown with chemical fertilizers and those sprayed with pesticides.

2. Any food that has been perverted with any kind of dangerous chemical additives and/or artificial processing.

3. Refined white flour and all products made from it.

4. Refined white sugar and all products made from it.

5. Salt and foods with salt added.

6. All fried foods, especially deep-fat frying.

7. Commercial cereals — all dry and cooked cereals that have gone through a long sterilizing chemical additive process; all cereals that have been fumigated with preservatives.

8. White rice and pearled barley.

9. Processed cheese.

10. Delicatessen foods which have salt or chemicals.

11. Chocolate in any form.

12. Hydrogenated Foods — Read the labels on peanut butter, margarine (of whatever kind, including corn, safflower or oil), and any other manufactured fats. If these are designated "hardened" or "hydrogenated" they are unfit to eat. All hydrogenated fats are almost pure cholesterol and would require a body heat of 300 degrees to be digested. Normal human body temperature is only 98.6 degrees — so these hydrogenated foods are indigestible.

To lengthen thy life, lessen thy meals.
Who is strong? He that can conquer his bad habits.
— Ben Franklin

"Living under conditions of modern life, it is important to bear in mind that the preparation and refinement of food products either entirely eliminates or in part destroys the vital elements in the original material."
— U.S. Dept. of Agriculture

The more natural the food you eat, the more radiant health you will enjoy and you will be better able to promote the higher life of love and brotherhood.
— Patricia Bragg

B. Meat & Fish — ("No-No Foods" continued)

1. Ham, bacon, luncheon meats, corned beef, hot dogs — all of which are preserved with high concentrations of inorganic sodium (salt) solutions and other harmful preservatives.

    (NEWS FLASH!!! — As this manuscript is being readied for the printer, a front page AP story reveals evidence that nitrite, a widely used preservative in smoked and processed meat and fish, combines with amines in the stomach to form a cancer-causing chemical which is transmitted through the blood-stream to various parts of the body. The lungs are particularly susceptible to cancer from this chemical, called nitrosamine. This research has just been completed by a team of doctors, University of Nebraska's Eppley Institute for Cancer Research.)

2. Smoked meat and fish.

3. Fish from inland waters which are diseased and suffering from the effects of pollutions that flow from civilization.

4. Pork is generally eliminated from the diet by most nutritionists, because this animal is often infected with a dangerous parasite called trichinosis. Pork is also very high in cholesterol content.

5. Most commercial meats have been injected with two highly toxic drugs — one to make the animal add weight, and one to make tough meat tender. Try to check the source of your meat supply, and find one where the meat is free from these dangerous drugs.

C. Seafood

1. Oysters, shrimp, crabs, lobsters and other shellfish that are caught too near outlets of city raw sewerage and other pollutants.

2. Seafood that has been sprayed with chemicals to give it a longer shelf life.

3. For safety, it is recommended that you confine your seafood eating to deep sea varieties that do not at any time inhabit coastal waters, because most coastal waters have become contaminated. (See Page 61 — "Select Your Seafood")

D. Beverages

1. Alcohol in any form.

2. Coffee and Tea.

3. Soft drinks and Cola drinks.

4. Chocolate drinks.

5. Fluoridated Water — If your city water has been fluoridated, don't drink it! Get yourself a home distiller and make
your own pure distilled water.

> (NOTE: We nutritionists highly condemn the practice
> of adding inorganic fluorides — a waste byproduct of
> the great aluminum companies — to the water in order
> to reduce tooth decay in young children. Any possible
> decrease in tooth decay is only temporary, and teeth
> become brittle and can give plenty of trouble later on.
> Research has proved that inorganic fluorine is one of
> most vicious and dangerous chemicals. There is much
> evidence that over a period of years the cumulative
> effect of drinking fluroidated water will endanger such
> organs as the heart, lungs, liver and kidneys. For the
> full story on fluoridation read my book, **"The Shocking
> Truth About Water."**)

DON'T SIMPLY "EAT WHAT AGREES WITH YOU"

Invariably, whenever nutrition is the topic of conversation in
a group of people, someone will boast, "I don't need to know one
thing about nutrition. I simply eat what agrees with me — and I
am in perfect health."

I can honestly say that I have buried most of these people. Just
because they were born with an exceptionally strong digestive
system, they thought they were indestructible. Poor, misguided
humans, thinking that they could stuff any kind of "food rubbish"
into their bodies and get away with it.

As far as food is concerned, such people carry their brains in
the taste buds of their mouths. "Trash" food may agree with
their taste — but not with their wonderful body chemistry.

> **The human body is a marvelous mechanism that
> will withstand a great deal of abuse — up to a
> point. But if you continue to abuse it and refuse
> to heed its warning signals, you will destroy it!**

So don't be confused by the person who rejects nutrition and
tells you, "Eat what agrees with you." This is the most deadly
advice you could accept about what to eat.

DON'T LET UNQUALIFIED PEOPLE CONFUSE YOU

Conversations on a city bus indicate how widespread is the confusion about nutrition. One day I overheard one woman telling another how poisonous onions were. Another time a woman was explaining how she cured her husband of the flu by feeding him chicken-noodle soup and chicken-rice soup.

Neither of these women has any qualifications or training whatsoever to make them authorities on nutrition.

Whenever anyone starts to tell you how healthful this or that food is, or how unhealthful it may be, ask yourself: What qualifications does this person have to be discussing nutritional science? What training has he/she had in biochemistry?

Don't heed unqualified advice.

DON'T LET THE AMATEUR NUTRITIONIST CONFUSE YOU

It is said that a little knowledge is a dangerous thing. And I believe this to be true.

People read a few books on diet and nutrition, hear a few lectures — and suddenly they are telling everyone they meet how to eat for health. I have heard these unknowledgeable amateur "experts" give some very wild and unscientific advice to suffering humans.

For example, one of these amateur nutritionists asserted that a mixture of olive oil, apple juice, lemon juice and vinegar would cause a person suffering with gallstones to pass the stones. This same man held forth about certain herbs that would cure this and that disease, and how certain foods would give one virility and sex power.

Don't be confused by this kind of advice.

SEEK PROFESSIONAL ASSISTANCE

If you are sincerely interested in proper nutrition go to your Health Food Store, purchase several books on nutrition and read them thoroughly. It is best to get nutritional advice from a professional rather than an amateur.

By reading several books on natural nutrition you will get a basis for comparison. Read each book carefully, and take from it the vital information that appeals to your intelligence.

As I said before, don't expect to find 100% agreement among these nutritionists as to the best diet of natural foods. Some will advocate a vegetarian diet, some a mixed diet, some a raw food diet, and so on. You will probably have to experiment with two or all of the various natural food diets to find the one — or a combination of several — best suited to your own body chemistry.

But remember, all these nutritionists agree that the first step is to eliminate all devitalized foods from your diet. Then you are ready to start on a program of proper nutrition.

Check back over the "No-No" List of what not to eat. Now let's have a look at the various natural food diets, so you may select what to eat for good health.

THE MACROBIOTIC DIET

Today many people follow the macrobiotic diet (from **makros** meaning "long" and **bios** meaning "life"), advocated by the late Japanese author George Ohsawa, who wrote many abstruse books on ancient Oriental diet and medicine. He was the principle proselytizer for macrobiotics in Europe and the U.S.A.

In macrobiotics, calories do not count. Neither does scientific nutritional balance.

"The only nutritional rules we discard are the modern ones," states Elaine Mensoff, 21, who cooks for a Boston macrobiotic group.

Macrobiotics concerns itself with those ancient complementary and opposite forces **yin** and **yang**, into which everything in the world is divided, including food. Sugar and most fruits, for example, tend to be very **yin**, while meats and eggs tend to be very **yang**.

The trick is to balance one's menus to maintain a 5-to-1 proportion of **yin** to **yang**. Since brown rice in itself contains this ratio, it is the principle food of the diet. I know people who follow this macrobiotic diet, who say that they have lived on brown rice exclusively for as long as thirty days.

Many qualified, university educated, biochemist nutritionists feel that the macrobiotic diet can be dangerous. To cite an example, five years ago 24-year-old Beth Ann Simon died after losing 50 pounds during nine months of an almost exclusive diet of only whole grain cereals, following Macrobiotic Regimen No. 7. Although this diet No. 7 is prescribed for special healing purposes and is intended to be followed for only 10 days at a time, other fatal cases of malnutrition as well as scurvy have been traced to it. Their **yin-yang** balance notwithstanding, brown rice and whole grain cereals alone are deficient not only in protein but also in valuable Vitamins A and C.

Most macrobiotics, as Ohsawa's followers call themselves, try to follow his other nine diets, which are graduated from six to minus three, including increasing amounts of fish and organically grown vegetables, along with brown rice. In actual practice, a good many younger macrobiotics also eat meat.

Michel Ahehsera, author of the cookbook recommended by the Whole Earth Group, explains, "Meat finds its way into the Zen macrobiotic diet simply as a concession to man's sensual desires."

Macrobiotics, like other panaceas, can be many things to many people. Some think it confers superhuman strength. But many macrobiotics use the diet to become less agressive and, above all, more spiritual.

"It's not the food that is important so much. It is the understanding. Through your food you are trying to attain the order of the universe," state many sincere macrobiotic enthusiasts.

Naturally, as a biochemist nutritionist I went to macrobiotic lectures and restaurants to investigate just what this type of diet consisted of. As an open minded researcher, I read all the books on the subject, and went to the homes of people who follow this way of eating.

First, I found that the macrobiotic diet lacked raw fruit and vegetables. One salad which they served me at a restaurant looked as though it had been through a washing machine, but I was told that this is the way they fix salads whenever they do eat them, which is not often.

Second, I found the macrobiotic diet saturated with inorganic sodium chloride. Since I have not used salt or eaten salty foods for many, many years, the taste buds of my mouth rejected the food. I could only taste it, but not eat it.

I am not trying to call the macrobiotic diet good or bad. It just has no appeal to me, and goes against all my principles of proper nutrition.

Now, if you read the books on this subject and it appeals to your intelligence, go on this macrobiotic diet. Nothing beats a trial but a failure. **This book is being written to help you help yourself to proper nutrition! The last thing I want to do is to confuse you!** As I stated at the start, my purpose is to present you with factual information on natural food diets, and to give you the benefit of my own research in the field of nutrition. You and you alone must accept or reject this macrobiotic diet or any other of the diets advocated by the various schools of natural nutrition.

THE RAW FOOD DIET

I honestly believe that every sincere student of nutrition at one time or the other decides to live exclusively on an all raw food diet. I admire them greatly for I, too, lived exclusively on a strict raw food diet for two years.

I was under the supervison of a famous advocate of this diet, Dr. Eugene Christian. I started following this diet with zest and enthusiasm, feeling that I was living on the perfect food for man — all raw foods.

Within two years, I dropped 25 pounds of weight, and lost much of my athletic strength, endurance and ability. I was hungry all the time, no matter how many avocados, nuts, seeds, raw fruit and vegetables I ate. It was a deep, unsatisfied hunger which could not be appeased by this strict raw food diet.

So, after two years on this raw food diet, I added cooked foods to my meals. I returned to normal weight, and again took up my athletic activities.

On the other side of the question, I have met people who have lived and thrived on an all raw food diet. Many raw fooders have told me that by following this diet they have defeated the worst heart conditions and other terminal degenerative diseases. A friend of mine in Hollywood, California, who is now in his late eighties, had a terrific heart attack fifty years ago. He was given two months to live. He went on the all raw food diet — and is enjoying perfect health today. I know a lady in Florida who had a deadly degenerative disease, with no hope of survival. She, too, went on the all raw food diet and is living in agelessness today.

In my long career as a nutritionist, I have met many outstanding advocates of the raw food diet — Dr. St. Louis Estes,

Dr. John Drews, Dr. Robert Welsh, Dr. & Mrs. John Richter, and many others. These men and women were dedicated to this philosophy of eating. But none of them lived to be 100 years of age, as they had anticipated.

In our researches among primitive peoples, neither Dr. Price nor I have ever found a race or tribe of healthy, long lived people who ate an exclusively raw food diet. Nor is there any factual evidence that races have lived on such a diet.

It is my personal belief that man at one time, eons ago before the ice age, lived in a perfect tropical environment where all conditons were ideal for living on a raw food diet.

But today we live in a filthy, poisoned, polluted and corrupt environment, pressured with tremendous stresses, strains and tensions. Even our best organically grown foods are deficient in many nutrients. That is why I also eat cooked foods and use natural food supplements to get extra nutrients into my body to withstand all the pressures which all of us must endure in this decaying super-civilization.

There are days when I eat fruit exclusively, especially in the summer when the fruit is naturally ripened by solar rays. There are days when I eat raw food exclusively, because I know this is a detoxifying diet. I think it helps to keep the bloodstream clean and wholesome. When watermelons are ripe and plentiful, I will live a week or more on watermelon and watermelon juice, as I believe that this flushing of the kidneys and liver is a superb way to move the toxic materials out of the body.

I often enjoy raw meals — such as a large tossed salad and nuts, or sun-dried apricots soaked overnight in pineapple juice. Living a strenuous and vigorous physical life as I do, I have learned by experience what to eat in both raw and cooked foods to sustain me with the greatest amount of vitality.

It is my personal opinion, based on observation and experience, that there are some people who are adaptable to an exclusively raw food diet, while others — like myself — are not. Again, you and you alone can discover to which category you belong. If the idea of a raw food diet appeals to you, by all means try it out. The reaction of your own body chemistry will give you the answer.

_____

The best way to lengthen life is to avoid shortening it.

THE VEGETARIAN DIET

The strict vegetarian diet consists of raw fruit, raw vegetables, cooked fruit and vegetables, whole grains, nuts, seeds, and dried fruits such as dates, figs and apricots.

I know countless vegetarians the world over who enjoy superior health on this diet. Here in the U.S. there are millions who have lived happily on a vegetarian diet for sixty years or more.

My friend Dr. John Harvey, of the famous Battle Creek Sanatarium, followed a strict vegetarian diet and lived a healthy life into his late nineties. Dr. John Maxwell, of Chicago, lived to be 103 — and for 80 of those years adhered strictly to the vegetarian regime. Charles Pierce, the slant board king, lived to be nearly 100 on a vegetarian diet. I climbed Mt. Hollywood with him on his 94th birthday. These are only a few examples of vegetarians who have lived long, healthful lives. They were enthusiastic followers of the strict vegetarian diet, and it worked splendidly for them. It is doing the same for many people today. I know a medical doctor, for example, who is forty years old but looks thirty. He has eaten an exclusive vegetarian diet for twenty years.

There is also the lacto-vegetarian, who adds dairy products and eggs to his diet. In my world travels I have found many people in a most healthful condition from following this diet.

In England especially you find a great number of both types, vegetarians and lacto-vegetarians. There is an English Vegetarian Society which has been active for more than 150 years. In London and other cities of England there are well known vegetarian restaurants, famous for their cuisine.

In working out your own nutritional program, you may wish to follow the example of these many satisfied and healthy vegetarians. To repeat, the selection of the diet best suited to your health needs must be determined by you and your own body chemistry.

THE MEAT DIET

The argument between vegetarians and meat eaters has been going on for many, many years. Both have strong points in favor of their systems of diet.

In recent years, however, even the most ardent meat eaters usually included other foods in their diet. As previously noted,

Prof. Robert McCracken, UCLA anthropologist, considers man's natural diet to be meat and fruit. Now more and more nutritionists — especially in the commercial group — are advocating large amounts of meat three times a day as a source of protein, especially in connection with the popularized all-protein reducing diet.

A doctor has even come out with a book stating that an exclusive meat diet is the perfect diet for man. He says that man is a carnivorous animal and has no need for any foods other than meat, including the fat.

I am well acquainted with this book, especially through people who have come to me for help after following its author's directions with disastrous results. Three men had suffered strokes from the excessive cholesterol that had accumulated in their arteries from this diet heavy in saturated animal fat. Several women who had followed this exclusive meat diet — which the author states "is the only diet that will get you thin and keep you thin" — came to me in serious condition from such a one-sided diet.

Just as man cannot live by bread alone, he cannot live by meat alone. **Meat is high in uric acid and in cholesterol content, both of which can be harmful to the human body in large quantities.** This is especially true today when so many people lead such sedentary lives.

Physical activity is required to burn up cholesterol as energy and to eliminate toxic uric acid. At my athletic club I can tell from the sweat of a person if he is a heavy meat eater. A putrid odor comes from the body, especially the feet and under the arms. Although unaware of it, most heavy meat eaters have a chronic case of halitosis. Their urine has a strong stench.

I agree that modern man evolved from meat-eating ancestors. But our forebears had to engage in strenuous physical activity in order to survive. Also, there is no evidence that they lived on an exclusive meat diet.

I must always come back to the researches by Dr. Price and by me among primitive peoples who have perfect health. These expeditions, as I have already mentioned, included research among Eskimos and Laplanders in the frigid north, where they live on an almost exclusive diet of reindeer meat. They are healthy people, free of cancer, arthritis and other diseases. Their environment and way of life determines their diet. Reindeer meat is lean — not streaked with fat like our commercially raised animals — and supplies the protein so necessary to keep humans warm and active in that cold climate.

Among primitive tribes in moderate and warm climates, however, neither Dr. Price nor I found any exclusive meat eaters. There were many who included meat, fish, eggs and poultry in their native diets — but there was always an abundance of other natural foods, such as raw fruits and vegetables, to balance the intake of meat.

Bernarr Macfadden, the "**father of physical culture**" with whom I was associated for many years, was this type of meat eater — and he was even parachuting from planes in his late eighties. I know many, many meat eaters who have lived long, energetic lives. Some of my meat-eating friends lived in robust health for 100 years or more.

Such people eat meat in moderation, and always balanced with other natural foods. My own advice to my health students, who wish to include meat in their diet, is to eat meat not more than three times a week.

If you eat animal protein, it is my contention that fish, organically raised turkeys and chickens have the least amount of toxins. Next come veal and lamb. Beef would take the last place. Many qualified nutritionists believe that the vital organs of the animal are superior in nourishment to the muscle meats. Brains, liver, tripe and sweetbreads are rich in nutrients.

To eat meat or not to eat meat — that is the question which you must decide for yourself. Acquaint yourself with both sides of the question, and study each side carefully. If you have a problem with cholesterol, uric acid or high blood pressure, then a vegetarian, salt-free diet should be more ideal until you reach a more normal status.

Many people go throughout life committing partial suicide — destroying their health, youth, beauty, talents, energies, creative qualities. Indeed, to learn how to be good to oneself is often more difficult than to learn how to be good to others.
— **Paul C. Bragg**

Now I see the secret of the making of the best persons, it is to grow in the open air, and eat and sleep with the earth.
— **Walt Whitman**

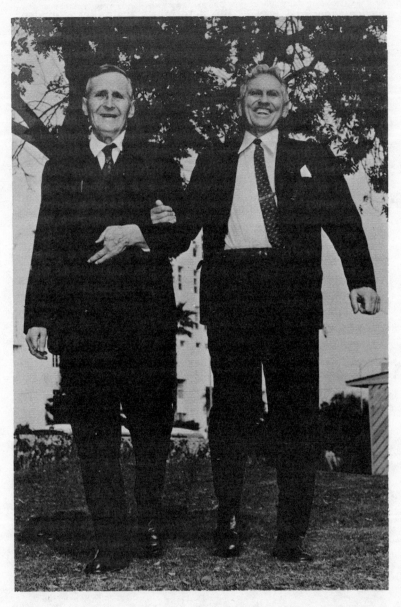

Roy D. White, left, a youthful 108, enjoys a healthy, active life — Here he starts on a five-mile walk with his friend, Paul C. Bragg.

THE "FOOD COMBINATION SYSTEM" DIET

There are some noted advocates of a dietary system based on "correct food combinations" — i.e., not mixing starches with proteins, etc. Dr. John Tilden, one of the really great nutritionists of our time, believed in the food combination theory — to eat all your starches at one time, all your proteins at another time, all your bulk foods at another, and so on. So did Dr. William Howard Hay of the famous Sun-Diet Sanatarium located in upper New York state.

Personally, this theory does not appeal to me. Eating is one of the greatest pleasures in life, and for me a system of non-mixing would appear to take a lot of pleasure out of one's diet unnecessarily. Also, I feel that it would make for confusion, as the average person would have to have the food combination book at the table at every meal to assure himself that he was eating the correct combination. The same would hold true in the kitchen for the person preparing the food. And think of the difficulty when traveling!

As I said, however, there are a number of qualified nutritionists who are ardent followers of the food combination system. Several of these were in the group of research doctors, dentists, biochemists and nutritionists with whom I went a few years ago into the baboon country of the African jungles to study the eating habits of this intelligent animal.

The baboon is really the king of the jungles. The mighty lion, who is supposed to bear that title, keeps his distance from the powerful vegetarian baboon.

Time after time during our observations of the eating habits of a tribe of baboons, we would see these strong, healthy animals holding a strictly protein food in one hand and a strictly starch food in the other, alternately taking a big bite of each.

After we returned to the States, I had dinner one evening with the food combination advocates who had been on this trip. I noticed that they had left that theory behind in the African jungles.

But let me repeat myself, if the food combination system of eating appeals to your intelligence, by all means try it. Study the books carefully, and if possible hear some lectures on the subject. It might be just the right thing for your digestion. It might be the answer to your nutritional problems. What the mind can conceive and believe, it can achieve!

THE "DON'T EAT" DIETS

"Don't Eat" diets come and go in infinite variety. Most of these are short-lived fads.

However, there are a few hardy perennials. One of these is: "Don't eat garlic, onions, cabbages, radishes and cauliflower, because these are sex stimulants."

In my opinion, if these foods really stimulated the sex desire and made it stronger, these vegetables would be raised by the millions of tons. Again I say test these vegetables and see what effect they have on your own body. You are the one eating them, and you should pass the final judgment whether they are to form a part of your diet.

Another diet expert, who is a strict vegetarian, states: "Don't eat honey. It's food for an animal, because a bee is an animal."

If you feel this is true about honey, then you will be able to survive very well without honey. If you want to eat it, remember that honey is a concentrated sugar and should be used with extreme moderation.

I have visited many strong, healthy, beautiful primitive people who do eat honey, and it surely has increased their energy.

But it's what you believe. You are the court of final judgment as to what you are going to eat or not eat.

THE MIXED DIET

During the past 65 years, I have seen many people come into a nutritional consciousness. Most of them, regardless of the many diets with which they experimented, finally end up — as I did — eating a mixed diet.

This diet includes raw fruit and vegetables, cooked fruit and vegetables, nuts, seeds, sun-dried raisins, dates, figs and apricots . . . several times a week adding fish, chicken, turkey, lamb and some beef to the menu.

My great friend Jack LaLanne — one of the country's finest physical training experts, as millions know who follow his TV program — has experimented with many diets. But today his diet consists of fresh raw vegetables and fruit, nuts, seeds, cooked vegetables, fish and poultry. In his middle fifties, Jack is probably the fittest man in the world — and looks it.

I will discuss the mixed diet of natural foods in more detail on following pages. But right now I would like to digress for a moment and theorize.

THE EVOLUTION OF NUTRITION

I have no factual evidence on the evolution of nutrition. I am only theorizing. But this is my honest belief after years of experimenting with every well-known so-called health diet.

I believe that man began life in a tropical paradise with an abundance of fruit and nuts. Along with this perfect food, all other environmental conditions were perfect. He lived in a warm climate where he wore no clothes, and therefore he exposed his body to the energizing solar rays of the sun. He slept on the ground under the sky, and not in a house where the oxygen is always limited. He was forced to do vigorous physical exercise. He had to climb trees to get his food. He had to walk miles to search for the different varieties of food.

Best of all, there were no pressures, tensions or stresses exerted upon his nervous system. The use of money was unknown. He had no taxes to pay, no electric, phone or gas bills. The only transportation he had was a pair of strong legs. He had no calendars, no clocks. He lived in agelessness — as I am endeavoring to do in this poisoned world!

Then the climate changed. The ice age came, and man was forced to eat any kind of food for his survival. The tropical paradise was covered with ice and snow, so he had to flee to a place where he could live and eat.

He then became a hunter. Modern anthropologists continue to find caves where primitive man left many bones of the animals he had eaten to survive. Man has been eating meat for an extremely long, indefinite period of time. Over these many years he has developed the digestive juices and the enzymes to assimilate meat.

Human nutrition, in my opinion, has thus evolved from the original ideal diet of fruit and nuts in an ideal environment, through various stages of environmental and consequent dietary changes, to present day man whose digestive system and body chemistry are best adapted to a mixed diet of natural foods.

Although civilized man today lives in a polluted, artificial environment, he cannot survive on polluted, artificial food. These environmental and dietary changes have not been brought about by nature — they are man's own abominable creations. In order to survive the damaging environment which he has brought upon himself . . .

Man needs today more than ever a balanced, wholesome diet of the natural foods which the human body demands!

NUTRITION IN ACTION

"The proof of the pudding is in the eating" is a very true old adage.

That is why my researches in nutrition have taken me from teeming cities to lonely deserts, from steaming jungles to the frigid north, from the mountains of Mexico to coral islands of the Pacific. That is why I have tested many different diets.

My conclusions are based on my observations and studies of nutrition in action.

Everywhere I have found that natural foods build and sustain health, and that unnatural, devitalized foods destroy it. Let me give you an illustration.

Forty years ago I made an expedition into a very isolated and primitive part of Mexico. I made a research study on nutrition among the several thousand Mexicans living in this area.

The basic item of their diet was the **tortilla,** a flat, thin, unleavened corn cake made from whole grain, stone ground native corn (maize), baked in a stone oven. The rest of their diet included native beans, goat cheese, chili, avocado, fruit and vegetables (both raw and cooked), seafoods and a small amount of meat.

These were healthy people with great endurance. In examining their teeth and bodies, I found them free of disease and with only 2% tooth decay. There were few retarded children, and very few congenital cripples.

These Mexicans, living on the native foods of their natural environment were not only healthy and vigorous but also happy.

They went about their daily life in a leisurely manner, really enjoying living. The men were exceptionally fine horsemen, and both men and women were vigorous dancers. If you have ever seen the Mexican Hat Dance, you know what I am talking about.

Some years later this area was discovered by the travel agents of the U.S.A. and other countries. More and more hotels were built to accommodate the increasing tourist trade.

And in poured the devitalized food and beverages. The local people no longer fished and grew naturally organic gardens. They were all working in some branch of the tourist trade, and had no time to prepare their natural foods. With the money they earned they purchased refined, bleached chemicalized white flour to replace their stone ground corn **tortillas**. They bought pasteurized, processed cheese instead of the wholesome home-made goat cheese, and ate canned beans rather than home cooked. They poured cola and soft drinks into themselves, as well as commercial ice cream, candy, cakes, and sugary canned fruits instead of the fresh native fruit. Instead of fresh fish and meat, they ate canned fish, hot dogs and luncheon meats.

When I revisited this area almost forty years after my first research there, this once healthy community had become a sick one. Where there was no hospital forty years ago, there are now three hospitals, various clinics, medical doctors and specialists, and many dentists.

The civilized diet of death had killed off all the healthy people I had met on my first visit, and now the children, grandchildren and great-grandchildren have completely degenerated with the devitalized diet.

This is what I mean by nutrition in action. Don't let the ivory tower theorists — sponsored by the powerful commercial food interests — confuse you! Remember that as long as people get a balanced diet of wholesome, natural foods they live in health, and as soon as they eat the dead-foods their health starts to fail.

Life is a tragedy of nutrition.
    — Prof. Arnold Ehret

HEALTH in a human being, is the perfection of bodily organization, intellectual energy, and moral power.
    — T. L. Nichols, M.D.

Be proud you live a natural health life.
    — Patricia Bragg

THE "HEALING CRISIS"

With civilized man being fed this diet of death from infancy onward, what chance does he have for a healthy life? Is there any way to reverse the process?

Fortunately, the answer is yes — if you have the desire and the determination to carry it through. But don't expect an overnight miracle. Depending on your calendar age, it has taken you that many years to saturate your body with the toxic poisons of a dead-food diet. It will take time to de-toxify your body.

As I have already emphasized, the first thing you must do is to eliminate all the dead-foods from your diet, as well as all drugs — and that includes tobacco, alcohol and medications.

The next step is to select the natural food diet which you want to follow— and start on it at once!

The change will be gradual, perhaps not even noticeable at first, but slowly you will begin to "feel better"! Be patient! Given a chance, the body is self-healing and self-repairing! — and now you have Mother Nature on your side! You are no longer seeking palliatives to relieve symptoms . . . you are seeking to eliminate the basic cause of your health problems!

The time it will take for your body to rejuvenate itself depends upon how much toxic poisons must be flushed out. Don't expect this process to be always comfortable! You are going to have good days and bad days!

As the toxic poisons begin to leave your body and become replaced with healthful nutrients, you will go through what we Naturopaths call a "healing crisis". You are likely to feel miserable and weak, you may have diarrhea and fever. You will probably discharge a great deal of mucus through your nose, mouth and bowels.

Don't be alarmed! What is happening is perfectly natural. As soon as you changed your unhealthy eating and living habits for a health-building program, you started to build your vital force and your recuperative power. You have now reached the crucial point when your vital force has become strong enough to take command and get rid of the toxic trash you have accumulated in your body for years. You are, at this point, on nature's operating table!

This "healing crisis" may last a day or a week or more —

again depending upon the amount of accumulated toxins that must be eliminated.

When it is past, you will begin to feel like a new person — as many people say, "reborn". You will not have another such crisis if you adhere faithfully to your health regime. There may be occasional "bad days" for a while, as hidden pockets of toxins are rooted out. But once the big crisis is over, you are "over the hump" on your road to health.

Let us now discuss some important guideposts to follow as you travel this Road to Radiant Health.

FASTING DETOXIFIES THE BODY!

While you are going through the major detoxification of your body during the "healing crisis", Mother Nature herself will force you to fast. The only food your stomach will accept will be fruit juice or distilled water.

This is as it should be. All the vital force, all the resources of your body are needed for the healing process!

In fact, from the point of view of natural healing, what is commonly called "illness" is actually nature's attempt to detoxify the body by an enforced fast! No animal ever eats when sick or injured! All creatures have a built-in instinct to fast at such times.

Poor, befuddled man, however, seems to have had this instinct "educated" out of him. He has been told over and over again that, when sick or injured, he must eat "to keep up his strength." Tragically, the attempt to keep up a sick person's strength by eating has put many a one into an early grave! In hospitals, when an ill person's body absolutely refuses food, the usual procedure is to force feed intravenously. In my opinion, such intravenous forced feeding in many instances does irreparable harm, prolongs the illness and may cause death.

Hippocrates, the father of Natural Healing, stated definitely that — *"fasting is the cornerstone of body healing."* This was in 500 B.C. at his Sanatarium on the Isle of Cos in the Aegean Sea. This precept has certainly stood the test of time. Today, almost 2500 years later, fasting is an important part of therapy in the great Natural Healing Institutions of England and Europe.

When I was dying of T.B. at age 16 and went to Dr. Rollier's sanatarium in Switzerland, fasting was an important part of my recovery.

After my remarkable recovery through the Science of Natural Healing, I visited some of the great Fasting Institutions of Europe. Dr. Reidlin of Germany was an outstanding doctor who used therapeutic fasting as the basis of his nature cure. Arnold Ehret conducted a great fasting sanatarium in Switzerland. Sick people from all over the world came to him for his supervision in fasting, and his cures seemed like miracles.

All the early Hygienic doctors in Europe and America used fasting as the basic of nature cure. When I first started in practice as a Naturopathic doctor I worked with the famous Bernarr Macfadden at his Natural Healing Institutions, where fasting was the basis of the treatment. Among the many other noted Natural Healers who have used therapeutic fasting with great success are Dr. William Howard Hay, Dr. Henry Lindlar, Dr. Frank McCoy, and Dr. John Tilden.

I have been fasting people therapeutically for more than 60 years, and by now have probably supervised more fasts than any other living man. For 25 years I conducted a fasting Health Resort, to which thousands came. Each case was carefully supervised.

This firsthand knowledge forms the basis of my book, **"The Miracle Of Fasting"**, which has benefited many more thousands of people. Every day I receive letters from many parts of the world from people who have regained health by following this program of therapeutic fasting.

I also receive many queries from many people who have become confused by authorities on nutrition who are opposed to fasting and consider it harmful.

In personal conferences with some of these health experts who criticize fasting, I have asked for factual evidence to support their negative statements. To date, not one of these critics has been able to give me prima facie documentary evidence of adverse effects of therapeutic fasting. Often I ask, "Did you ever fast in your life?" Usually I receive some such reply as, "Yes. Several years ago I had a battle with pneumonia and I did not eat food for nine days. The only thing that passed my lips was water."

Little do such people realize that this fasting had a direct connection with their recovery. But that is the way Mother Nature operates . . . when you won't fast yourself, she takes you in her capable hands and saves your life by a forced fast.

I find that the critics of therapeutic fasting have never studied the subject, and are therefore totally unqualified to pass on its merits. Everyone has a perfect right to his opinion on fasting — but opinions have no meaning. It is factual documentary evidence that counts. And the preponderance of factual evidence is that fasting is man's greatest natural healer.

In this connection, it is interesting to note that all the great religions — Christianity, Judaism, Buddhism and Mohammedanism — practice fasting at various times of the year for purification of body and mind. Surely if fasting were detrimental, these great faiths would have abandoned it long ago.

A word of caution: I do not advise my students to go on long fasts unless they are expertly supervised. There are Health Spas that will supervise fasts in many parts of the world.

It is my own practice to fast one 24-hour period every week. On Mondays I eat my usual meals . . . but from Monday night to Tuesday evening I eat nothing. During this time I drink only distilled water. I give my digestive and elimination system a complete rest. I skip breakfast and lunch, then eat my usual dinner Tuesday evening.

Several times each year I take a longer "super" fast. I go on a complete distilled water fast for an entire week. This means no vegetables, juices, or fresh fruit. It is a complete fast. And it works wonders in keeping me fit! Remember my book, **"Miracle of Fasting"**, goes into all details about fasting.

GARLIC — "THE POOR MAN'S PENICILLIN"

Nature not only prescribes fasting as a means of regaining health . . . this good mother also provides foods to keep us well.

Garlic, for example, is a natural antibiotic. Again, this is not a statement of opinion . . . but a statement of documented fact.

And again I must cite the good Dr. Rollier as the person who first made me aware of the healing properties of garlic. Fresh raw garlic, he said, is the killer of T.B. germs. And did we consume the garlic at his sanatarium in Switzerland! No respectable T.B. bugs could live in my body with all the garlic I ate!

Since those days at Dr. Rollier's sanatarium, where I regained life and health, I have consumed literally tons of garlic. And I am free of the illnesses that plague so many of my fellow humans. My blood pressure is that of a man in his twenties. I owe much of my ageless health to garlic.

I have researched the crowded Arab cities of North Africa, where humans live in the worst filth, squalor and poverty I have ever seen. But with all that filth, you find no infectious diseases as you do in clean, hygienic America.

I asked an African doctor why, with all this terrible dirt and squalor, these people do not die of many infectious diseases.

And the good doctor smiled and said, **"These people eat the greatest bacteria and virus antibiotic in the world — garlic!"**

Because of its antibiotic properties, garlic has become known as **"The poor man's penicillin."**

So many people have been influenced by the anti-halitosis ads and commercials that they refuse to eat garlic "for fear of offending."

Isn't it much better to let your friends and acquaintances smell garlic on your breath than to infect them with a cold virus? And, of course, if your friends and acquaintances would be so health-minded as to eat garlic, too, no one would be aware of any breath odor.

To me, the smell of garlic is a good, healthy odor. And the taste of garlic adds zest to many foods. The French, world famous for their cuisine, use garlic in almost everything.

Judging from my mail, a great deal of confusion is being created lately by diet experts who warn against the eating of garlic and a long list of other natural foods. When you hear or read such unnatural advice, check the source. Is this authority qualified on this subject? Has he/she studied the science of natural foods? What documented facts are used to support this adverse opinion? Is it merely a personal or prejudiced reaction?

"Wisdom does not show itself so much in precept as in life — a firmness of mind and mastery of appetite."   **— Seneca**

Habits of rapid eating are most harmful, and must be overcome. Quietness and Cheerfulness at meals is most essential.   **— Oliver Wendell Holmes**

Are these diet experts acting as spokesmen for the commercial food industry?

Let your intelligence and your desire for good health be your guides. Find out for yourself if garlic adds zest to your food and your physical vigor.

WHOLE GRAIN FOODS ARE HEALTHFUL

Another important part of the natural diet which saved me from death with T.B. was freshly stone-ground rye flour, grown in a fertile valley of Switzerland. This was the isolated Loetschental Valley, which had a 900-year record of having no doctors and no dentists. The people there enjoyed an unusually high grade of health.

It was also at the Rollier Sanatarium in Leysin, Switzerland that I read a remarkable book on the value of whole grains by Sylvester Graham, one of the great pioneers in America on natural foods. Graham flour is named after this man.

After my recovery, I travelled all over rural Europe studying the food habits of the people of different countries. In Germany I ate the coarse, dark rye bread known as pumpernickel. I ate the coarse black rye bread of Austria-Hungary. And on my tour through Russia I ate the black bread of Russia.

All these people in the rural areas of these countries were strong, energetic and long-lived. Among these hearty people I found none of the miseries — such as constipation, stomach ailments, colds, heart trouble and so on — that plagued urban populations even then and most people throughout the Western world today.

While I was in Siberia in the frigid cold of winter, I thrived on the same diet that kept these people healthy and vigorous — coarse black rye bread, beet soup, cabbage, carrots and natural sheep cheese. They did extra heavy manual labor all during the long winter, lumbering and mining. After a day of hard work they ate their simple meals, then spent several hours dancing, often leaping five or six feet off the floor. They loved to sing, too, and had rich, strong voices. It was such men as these who composed the famous Cossack Cavalry.

Whole grain oats form a basic part of the Scotch diet — and what rugged, vigorous, bonny men and women are those Highland Scots! They, too, are strenuous dancers . . . it takes a lot of energy to dance a real Highland Fling. They are happy, fun-loving, kindly, sweet people . . . and also intrepid fighters. When Scotch soldiers in World War I came to battle in their traditional kilts, they were at first ridiculed for wearing skirts . . . but their strength and daring fighting skill soon won them the epithet of "Ladies from Hell".

Whole grain barley has also stood the test of time as a food for centuries. It has been a staple of Mid-Eastern diet since Biblical times.

I have previously discussed the importance of whole grain corn in the Mexican diet. As a matter of fact, the records of the spanish conquistadores, which have been preserved in the archives of Spain and which I have studied with great care, show that this native corn (maize) was also important in the diet of the highly advanced civilizations of the Aztecs and Mayans centuries ago. The Spaniards reported that these races were healthy, powerful people, free of disease. They found no bald-headed men, no retarded or congenitally crippled children. There were no insane persons, no premature ageing, no decayed teeth. Their bodies, both young and matured, were things of beauty.

These ancient peoples of America were also highly developed in intelligence. They were scientific astronomers, architects, mathematicians and agriculturists. They developed the potato, many varieties of squash, beans, red peppers, cheese and corn as we know these today.

The healthiest and most long-lived people in the world today are the Hunza nation. The documentary motion picture of these remarkable people, taken by Renee Taylor, shows them stone-grinding their whole grains and making this flour into bread.

When I joined the famous health man, Bernarr Macfadden, at the turn of this century to work with him as associate editor of the **Physical Culture Magazine,** Macfadden strongly advocated the eating of whole wheat bread. He served this famous Mac-fadden bread in all his health restaurants.

Macfadden also developed a healthful cereal by soaking whole-wheat kernels overnight, then steaming them until they popped open. He would serve this with honey . . . and it was as delicious as it was nutritious. During the depression of the 1930's he opened penny restaurants all over America, where he served a large bowl of this steamed wheat and honey for one penny. Thousands upon thousands were saved from starvation by this simple meal.

Macfadden lived to be in his late eighties . . . a long time for a man who, like myself, was given a death sentence with T.B. in his youth. For more than sixty years of his life, his whole-grain bread and his steamed whole-wheat cereal were key items in his diet. During the years of my association with him, I never knew him to suffer any kind of illness.

My children were reared on this same steamed whole-wheat cereal and bread made of 100% stone-ground grain. Their teeth never had cavities, and they never missed a day in school on account of illness.

It is only since the refining process in making commercial flour was introduced that many human ills have become prevalent. The refining, bleaching process eliminates all the natural nutrients, vitamins and minerals from the grain and changes it from a life-giving, health-building food into a dead-food.

The same is true of rice. The rice eating peoples of Asia have survived hardily for thousands of years with natural brown rice as their basic food. But when they start using civilized white rice, which has lost its coat that contains the B-Complex and other important vitamins, minerals and nutrients, their health degenerates. Here in Hawaii, where this book is being written, there are many Orientals among the population. The preponderance of these people use devitalized white rice as the basic item of their diet. As a result, much of their money and time is spent on hospitals, clinics, doctors and dentists, because of sick bodies and decaying teeth.

So let me warn you again not to be confused by commercial diet experts who extol the nutritional virtues of dead cereals, refined white flour and refined white rice.

Try incorporating natural whole grain foods into your diet, and find out if these benefit you as they have others who now enjoy a healthful life.

"Our Prayers should be for a sound mind in a healthy body."
— Juvenal

Life is like a gun. It can be aimed in only one direction at a time.
Make your aim — health!
— Paul C. Bragg

WHAT ABOUT EGGS?

There are a great many pros and cons about the eating of eggs, with well qualified nutritionists and doctors on both sides and in the middle.

Eggs have been used for food by man since prehistoric days. The Chinese have been eating eggs for more than 6,000 years. All over the world, most people who can afford eggs eat them.

The very latest scientific research on eggs places this food at the top of the list for protein. This research asserts that eggs may be included in the diet of heart cases, because eggs — which contain cholesterol — also contain lecithin which is the antidote to cholesterol. The claim is made that the yolks are rich in Vitamin A, and that children who do not eat eggs may get rheumatoid arthritis but those who eat eggs are free of this disease.

Back again to the Rollier Sanatarium where my life was restored . . . my diet there included three fertile hard boiled eggs weekly. Dr. Rollier considered three eggs all that the human body should have within a week. In my diet today I do not average that many . . . but when my body chemistry tells me I need a few fertile eggs, I answer the call. I eat my eggs as they were served to me at the sanatarium — hard boiled, seasoned with chopped raw garlic and imported olive oil. (All Dr. Rollier's patients were given a tablespoon of good imported olive oil daily, because Dr. Rollier said it helped harden the gums.)

My good friend Bernard Shaw, the great writer, ate three eggs a week. He lived in good health into his late nineties, when a fall from a tree he was pruning hastened his death. Another good friend, Indian Princess Duprea, lived to the age of 115 and ate eggs every day of her long, healthy life.

Dr. John Maxwell, my vegetarian friend who lived to be 103, at three eggs weekly. In my world travels I have met many men and women over 100 years of age who have eaten eggs in moderation all their lives.

Such people, however, are particular about the kind of eggs they eat. Fresh eggs from healthy, fertile hens are correctly classified as natural food. A healthy hen, scratching for her own natural food, gets plenty of exercise and a diet properly balanced for her own body chemistry, which determines the quality of her eggs. By nature's way, a healthy hen lays one or perhaps two eggs daily — in the daytime. **"To bed with the chickens"** means asleep at dark. I often revert back to my early youth and farm life and go to bed at dark — but I'm always up at sunrise for I love the early morning for exercise, meditation and I find it the most peaceful time for writing.

The commercial "egg factories", however, which produce most of the eggs sold in supermarkets today, change natural, healthy hens into egg-laying machines by confining these poor creatures to rows of wire-mesh nests in a barracks-like structure which is artificially ventilated and artificially lighted 24 hours a day. Since it is never dark, the hens don't sleep . . . they just keep on laying eggs. They get no exercise, and are fed on commercial mixtures. They produce a great many more eggs — but what kind of eggs are these? The eggs of these poor, exhausted creatures are unfertile . . . the yolks are loaded with the residue of cholesterol which the hen would normally have used up as fuel if allowed natural exercise . . . and no doubt some toxins from these unhealthy hens could be passed on into their eggs.

It is because of these commercially produced eggs — which may be even further deteriorated by cold storage before reaching the supermarkets — that many cardiac specialists eliminate eggs from the diet of heart patients.

So, if you wish to include eggs in your diet, be sure to use fresh, fertile eggs from healthy hens.

SELECT YOUR SEAFOOD

Fresh, uncontaminated seafood is one of nature's most nourishing foods. It is excellent as a protein and as a source of Vitamins A, B and D, as well as organic iron, calcium and phosphorous. Saltwater fish contain more natural iodine than any known common food.

Today, however, you must exercise great care in the selection of your seafood. One of the worst crimes of civilization is the excessive pollution of our waters, not only with raw sewage and garbage but also with poisonous chemicals discharged by industrial plants. Our inland waters have become so polluted that fish are dying — and so are people who eat them. Fresh fish are safely edible only in isolated, protected areas.

Now the pollution extends into our coastal waters, contaminated by polluted rivers which empty into the oceans, as well as by rampage of waste into our harbors. One of man's principal sources of food since prehistoric days is thus becoming a source of poison.

A recent announcement by the Federal Food & Drug Administration disclosed the frightening fact that "one can of commercial tuna in every five it sampled contained poisonous mercury in excess of federal limits" in the 1970 tuna pack of approximately 864 million cans for domestic use.

If you are on a natural food diet, of course, you will not be eating canned (salted, preserved) tuna — but the canning process is not to blame for its mercury content. This poison was in the fish before it was caught! Tuna spawn and live in shoals along the coasts during the spring and summer, going out into deep water only during the winter months. Mercury discharged by industrial plants into rivers is carried to the sea and emptied into the shoals where it is absorbed by the tuna — probably through the gills when breathing as well as by its food which has also been contaminated by this poison.

A still later release by the FDA has revealed that a dangerous amount of mercury has also been found in swordfish. This prized fish inhabits both coasts of the United States.

Although I have seen no such report yet on salmon, this excellent food fish spawns in the headwaters of inland streams and could also become contaminated on its journey downriver to the sea.

Investigations will no doubt continue, after this book goes to print, so watch newspapers and health magazines for further reports.

Although the FDA has established what is designated as a "safe level" of mercury content, the point has been made by physicians that this poison can accumulate in the human body . . . so the continuous eating of fish with a "safe level" mercury content can build up to a dangerous content of this poison in your system.

As previously noted, shellfish such as oysters, shrimp, crab, lobsters and the like, which are taken near the outlets of polluted rivers, can be "hazardous to your health".

Ecologists are on the warpath to eliminate mercury, raw

sewage and other poisonous pollutants from our streams, rivers, lakes and coastal water. But the ecology crusaders are opposed by powerful industrial interests, and it is likely to be a very long time before civilized man cleans his own house.

So, aid the ecologists in their clean-up campaign . . . and in the meantime, determine the source of your seafood and select only deep sea fish from safe, uncontaminated waters.

So far, civilization does not appear to have contaminated many of the South Pacific waters. One place where I always enjoy seafood with a sense of safety is in New Zealand, a land which I have come to love very strongly. I have property there in an isolated section of the North Island . . . where, incidentally, the famous American author, Zane Grey, had his fishing headquarters and made many of his noted moving pictures documenting the catching of all kinds of big fish.

Near my place is a native Maori village, whose people live exclusively on seafood and other native foods. They have beautiful, powerful bodies, radiant health and keen, alert minds. And they are an unusually happy people.

Early explorers called New Zealand **"The Pacific Garden of Eden"**, because it was such a beautiful, healthy country and its native Maori people had such superb health and splendid physiques. They were totally without disease and showed no signs of premature ageing.

The basic native Maori diet was, and still is, food from the sea surrounding the two islands that form their country. Even today, in spite of the encroachment of the white man and his civilized diet of death, on my lecture tours in New Zealand I find many wonderfully healthy Maori among the people in my audiences. The Maori women are beautiful in face and form. The Maori men have great physical endurance and good minds, and many of them are leading lawyers and government executives.

Naturally, the breakdown of these fine native people comes when they depart from their natural seafood diet and eat the dead-foods of modern civlization. The effect is similar to that experienced by other native races and peoples contaminated by Western civilization.

Let us hope that the governments of New Zealand and other areas of the South Pacific will be sufficiently alert to protect their waters, both inland and coastal, from the plague of civilized pollution . . . and preserve their native treasure of health-giving seafood!

RIPE BANANAS ARE A PERFECT FOOD

The very first food a South Sea mother gives her child is a mashed banana, and from then on bananas form an important part of his lifelong diet. Here in Hawaii, where I am writing this book, there are 27 varieties of delicious and nutritious bananas . . . and I eat bananas daily, both because I like them and because I regard them as a splendid natural food.

Following the practice of the South Seas, the first food I gave my young babies was fresh, ripe bananas. As they grew up, one of the children's favorite health desserts was Bragg Baked Bananas. Here's the recipe:

Place 10 peeled bananas in a baking pan, and pour over them a cupful of fresh, pure orange juice. Add a tablespoon of honey, then another ½ cup of orange juice with a heaping teaspoon of arrowroot to thicken the sauce, and a dash of vanilla. Bake in an oven under low heat for 20 minutes until the bananas become soft to the touch of a fork — not mushy, just soft. Cool the dish, then chill it in the refrigerator before serving. It is delicious hot also.

My children loved it. And the bananas supplied their growing bodies with important vitamins, minerals and nutrients, and aided bowel elimination.

Bananas are one of the finest sources of organic potassium, and for this reason many heart specialists prescribe two bananas daily for patients on a salt-free diet.

I have fed bananas to ulcer patients who could tolerate no other food. The same with those suffering from colitis, who found bananas the only food they could eat without distress. Be sure the bananas are ripe before eating, then you get the full banana flavor.

Recently I have had inquiries from people who have become confused by references to the discovery of a substance called serotonin in bananas.

The authoritative Dorland's Medical Dictionary defines serotonin as **"a vasoconstrictor compound found in the serum of**

mammals.'' This means that it is a natural component of the blood of mammals, including humans, which the body chemistry utilizes when necessary to constrict small blood vessels, especially the arterioles (arterial capillaries). For example, when you are exposed to cold weather or in a cold room, the serotonin in your blood reacts to narrow the capillaries in your extremities — feet, hands, nose, ears — and thus restrict the circulation in those exposed areas, so that your inner body temperature will remain normal. This is a built-in protective reaction.

Since serotonin is a natural substance of human body chemistry, it cannot be considered harmful . . . and I personally have never had any adverse reaction from eating bananas (and I have consumed tons of them!), nor have I ever known anyone who has.

However, if you feel any unpleasant reaction such as abnormally cold hands or feet after eating a number of bananas, then restrict your banana quota to several a week.

In my own research and experience, I have found the banana to be one of the really perfect foods of man for both the well and the sick, when eaten fully ripened. When the peel of the banana is covered with brown spots, it is at its height of ripeness.

CITRUS IS A PRIME SOURCE OF VITAMIN C

The **"miracle healing"** quality of citrus fruit was discovered long before vitamins were. It was during the days of sailing ships, when even sailors who loved the sea feared to go on long ocean journeys because of the dread disease scurvy. On these long voyages, scurvy laid even the strongest men low, making them so weak they could not move a muscle. Entire crews were incapacitated, and thousands of sailors died from scurvy.

England was then ruler of the seas, but the invisible enemy scurvy threatened to sap her strength. Then it was that the great explorer Captain Cook, who discovered the Hawaiian Islands, made his greatest discovery of all — the connection between this dread disease and the diet which caused it. On voyages which lasted months and even years, the sailors lived on salted food and were deprived of fresh meat, vegetables and fruit.

The deficiency was found to be almost magically filled by eating fresh citrus fruit — limes, lemons, oranges — or drinking the juice. Within hours the extreme weakness, anemia and bleeding, spongy gums of scurvy disappeared. Since limes were the easiest to store aboard ship, this fruit became a requisite of the sailors' diet, and British sailors became known throughout the world as "limeys".

Centuries later came the discovery of vitamins, and the "miraculous" ingredient of citrus fruit that cured and prevented scurvy was found to be Vitamin C.

Today citrus fruits are so prevalent throughout most of the world, with the greatest quantity being produced in the U.S.A., that few people remember where they originated. The lime and orange are natives of Southeast Asia, the lemon of India, and the grapefruit — a comparative newcomer — is a cultivated version of the native shaddock of the American tropics (named for another English explorer, Captain Shaddock).

To me, citrus fruit can still be called a "miracle food". Vitality Vitamin C, of which it is the prime source, is a preventative not only of scurvy but of many other human ailments. Thousands of pediatricians (specialists in the care of infants and children) prescribe orange juice for their young patients. My children grew up eating oranges and grapefruit fresh from the trees in our Southern California garden.

These citrus eating children are not subject to colds and flu, and are not plagued with heavy mucus as some of their playmates are.

Grapefruit is exceptionally rich in Vitamin C, and it was in my own date groves in the California desert that I learned how to "beat the heat" with high amounts of Vitamin C supplied by grapefruit.

In the summertime the heat and humidity get almost unbearable in these irrigated date groves, and I found it very difficult to keep workers on the job. Then one day a new man applied for work in my grove, bringing a bag of grapefruit with him. He worked tirelessly, doing the work of any four of the other men — scampering up and down the ladders on the date palms, shoveling out irrigation ditches. Several times during the day he would pause long enough to take a grapefruit out of his bag and eat it.

This man was no ordinary worker, I discovered. He was a noted biochemist, who had come out to the California desert date country to test his theory that when a person sweats, he loses Vitamin C . . . and that he can easily "beat the heat" and retain his vitality under intense heat and humidity by keeping his body well supplied with this essential vitamin.

I entered wholeheartedly into this research project. I kept an ample supply of cooled grapefruit for my workers and placed a juicer at their disposal, so the men could eat the grapefruit or drink the juice. And what a change came over them, mentally and physically! Not only did they accomplish three and four times as much work as before, but they also joked and sang while they worked.

The young biochemist and I continued this research in the cottonfields of Imperial Valley, also in the California desert country, with the same miraculous results. The workers sweating wearily in the sun became refreshed and vigorous.

We studied the effect of Vitamin C on athletes in various sports, and found that it gave them more energy, endurance and stamina. Then I thought of the movie stars who work under the intense heat of powerful klieg lights, and again Vitality Vitamin C did the trick, enabling them to work longer under the bright, hot lights without becoming exhausted and short-tempered.

Chemically known as ascorbic acid, Vitamin C is often called **"the most needed vitamin"**. It is found in all the fluids and tissues of the body; it acts as a "cement" to hold the body cells together; it gives firmness to ligaments, cartileges, blood vessel walls, and even the matrix of the bones and teeth. It helps speed the healing of wounds!

Being water soluble, Vitamin C is not easily stored in the body but is excreted in the urine and perspiration. That is why it is necessary to provide your body with a continuous supply . . . and citrus fruit is a prime source of this essential vitamin.

DRINK VEGETABLE JUICES IN MODERATION

Although you receive the same nutritional value from citrus with either the whole fruit or the juice, this does not hold true in regard to vegetables.

Different vegetables supply the body with different vitamins, minerals and nutrients. For example, green beans are an excellent source of organic iron, while dried beans give excellent supplies of Vitamins B_1, B_2 and C, and organic phosphorous and copper. Mustard greens rate "excellent" in Vitamin A, Vitamin C and organic calcium, while mushrooms excel in providing Vitamin B , niacin and organic copper. (For a detailed table of food sources of vitamins and minerals, see my . . . **"Bragg Four Generation Health Food Cook Book".**)

All vegetables, however, supply two other essentials of proper nutrition — moisture and bulk. Although you may obtain many of the vitamins and minerals in vegetable juices, you do not get the necessary combination of moisture and bulk in your intestines for healthy elimination of waste, unless you eat the vegetables raw or properly cooked.

In the early 1920's when I visited Germany, live juice therapy was all the rage there. At that time all juices were made with a hand juicer. I purchased the distributorship for this juicer for the United States. I wrote a book on live juice therapy and gave lectures on this subject throughout the U.S.A.

In both my book and lectures, I stressed the point that one 6-ounce glass of mixed vegetable juices — such as carrot, beet, celery and parsley — was sufficient for one day's ration, and that the greater portion of vegetables in a natural health diet should be eaten. With the hand juicer, time and energy were required to squeeze 6 to 8 ounces of vegetable juice, and people who drank this amount gained valuable nutritional results!

But when the first electric juicer arrived on the market in 1937, health-minded people purchased them by the thousands. No longer was the difficult hand juicer necessary . . . in just a few minutes with the electric juicer, you could make several quarts of vegetable juice.

Health people went on a vegetable juice binge. They thought that, if a small amount of this juice is good for health, a gallon would mean greater health. They became vegetable juice drunkards. And the binge continues today. As I travel around the world on my lecture tours, I am finding more and more people who are turning yellow from drinking too much carrot juice. Yes, that's right . . . they look as though they had jaundice!

The body needs and can use only so much raw vegetable juice, regardless of the intake. The surplus is passed out by the kidneys. In the case of over-indulgence in carrot juice, the yellow pigment is not eliminated but is absorbed into the skin tissues.

I drink a 6-to-8-ounce glass of mixed raw vegetable juice three or four times a week. This amount I consider beneficial to my nutritional health. The rest of my vegetables — by far the greater portion — I eat raw or cooked. Raw carrots, beets and celery are especially good providers of moisture and bulk — and when eaten this way, the yellow pigment of the carrot is eliminated along with the bulk. Fresh juices are concentrated sugars and should be limited for they could throw your sugar-insulin balance off.

NATURAL FOOD SUPPLEMENTS

If you eat a well balanced diet of natural foods, why do you need food supplements?

Even if you eat the nutritionally best possible diet, it is my opinion — based on experience and study — that you do not obtain enough vitamins, minerals and trace minerals for vigorous health. Even in the best organically grown food there are nutritional factors missing. When foods are bought in the market, much of the fresh food has lost its vitamin content during the long shipping process from grower to consumer.

That is why I consider food supplements an important nutrient. I take them with my meals . . . including a multi-vitamin-mineral supplement, and 1200 I.U. of natural Vitamin E, B- Complex, Calcium, Vitamin A, and Vitamin C.

Be sure that you get natural food supplements from your Health Food Store. Keep away from the synthetic supplements. The same principles of nutrition apply in food supplements as in food itself.

From my mail, there seems to be current confusion about taking food supplements which contain both calcium and phosphorous, that such a combination is dangerous. This is false.

As a biochemist and nutritionist, I can definitely state that anywhere in nature, organic or inorganic, wherever you find calcium you will always find phosphorous as well. These two minerals are affinities, just as copper and iron are affinities.

I have been taking an organic calcium and phosphorous food supplement for many years with perfect results.

WHAT IS THE PERFECT DIET OF MAN?

Every sincere person who wants to eat for health, (freedom from pain and illness), for energy, endurance, youthful looks and

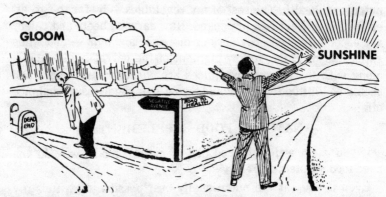

The choice of which road to take is up to the individual. He alone can decide whether he wants to reach a dead end or live a healthy, wholesome, long, active life.

feelings, is striving to find the perfect diet of man. This has been my quest for more than sixty years.

As yet, no perfect diet system has been discovered that provides perfect nutrition for everyone. Nutrition is a young science, and there is still a great deal to be learned about foods.

Again let me remind you what Dr. Price and I and other research workers have found when we studied the diet systems and habits of isolated primitive peoples. All of us agree that there are healthy people in many primitive places and many climates, and that none of them live on the same system of eating. There are healthy meat eaters, healthy vegetarians, and so on.

YOU MUST SELECT YOUR OWN PERFECT DIET

As you start studying the Science of Nutrition, you will find a wide variety of nutritionists and dieticians — some reliable, some not — advocating an equally wide variety of diets. Don't become confused! Weigh the evidence, and study your own body's reactions to different diets. You, and only you, can finally select the perfect diet for your own health.

I am a mountain climber, and I have climbed high mountains

in many parts of the world with vegetarians, fruitarians, raw fooders, mixed eaters. They were all fearless, strong, sturdy men and women. They were not confused about their diets. What they ate nourished and satisfied them.

They all had one thing in common. They ate no devitalized, de-nutritionized, devitamized and de-mineralized foods. Each ate the natural food diet which he/she had learned by experience was personally the most healthful for them.

And so let it be with you. In selecting your personal diet, read what the experts have to say. If it appeals to your intelligence, see what it does for you. No one in the world, no diet expert, can tell you how certain foods are going to react in your body. You must experiment with various systems of diet, and choose which one fits your nutritional needs. If one does not work, try another until you find the right one for you.

COMMUNICATE WITH YOUR BODY

Being an athlete and expending great amounts of energy, I have tried to create for myself a diet that would keep me in excellent health and have as little toxic material forming in my body as possible.

To do this, I have developed excellent communication with my body. There is no "communication gap" between my mind and my body chemistry.

As I have detoxified my body by regular weekly 24-hour fasts and occasional "super fasts" of 7 to 21 days, I have been able to add more fresh fruit and raw vegetables to my diet.

When I stopped fretting and worrying as to whether I was getting enough protein or not, I made my greatest advances in health building. I now realize that the body chemistry has the power to convert any food I eat into a protein. Little by little I lost my desire for meat, and seemed to enjoy nuts and seeds more.

"Govern well thy appetite, lest Sin surprise thee, and her black attendant Death."
— Milton

Ninety per cent of our disorders are due to errors in diet.
The majority eat more than is good for them.
— Sir Hy. Thompson, M.D.

But when my body communicates a need for meat or fish or eggs, I eat them.

You must develop a deep communication between food and your body chemistry.

> **It took me many years to discard the emotions when it came to eating. But eating is one thing about which you must not be emotional!**

Every day I go into consultation with my body chemistry and try to find out its needs. This is done on a non-emotional basis. One day it might tell me to fast on distilled water or to eat salads and fruits only, etc.

As you purify your body by discarding the "trash" foods, a great enlightenment comes. The "communication gap" between you and your body chemistry becomes bridged. You realize that your body needs nutrients to keep you alive, and that it knows what it needs. And you learn how to supply those needs.

MY OWN DIET IS VARIED

As I have stated, I have tried every type of natural dietetic system that has been offered. For myself, I believe that I have found the ideal diet for my body chemistry in a varied diet derived from that of the strong, healthy primitive people I have studied.

I have had to do a great deal of experimenting to find a diet which keeps me in agelessness . . . a diet which satisfies the taste buds of the mouth . . . a diet which keeps me energetic so that I can enjoy physical effort such as jogging, swimming, climbing mountains, playing tennis, hiking . . . a diet which keeps me mentally alert so that I am able to lecture and write articles and books.

The diet I have worked out for myself meets my needs. I don't expect it to be perfect for everyone else. We are all different in our nutritional needs.

It is my hope that this book will provide a channel to clear the confusion about nutrition, so that you can work out a diet for yourself which will satisfy your body needs.

Let food be your medicine, and medicine be your food. — **Hippocrates**

THE BODY MUST EARN ITS FOOD

It is my experience that proper exercise and proper nutrition must go hand in hand. I believe that the body must earn its food.

That is why I never eat breakfast. I have not eaten a regular breakfast for the past 65 years. I believe that eating breakfast is just a habit — and a bad health habit, at that. Sleeping does not earn one a hearty breakfast.

In the morning is the time my body craves physical activity and large amounts of oxygen. Here in my second home, Honolulu, Hawaii, where this book is being written, my program is to arise at 5 to 5:30 a.m. I do not force myself to arise this early, my body tells me it's time to get up and get active physically.

First I do my yoga exercises (standing on my head, etc.), then go out on the beach at Waikiki and jog. I love to jog and run. Then I take a swim and a period of abdominal exercises. A long walk in the sand to exercise my feet . . . and I return home after three hours of steady physical activity. When I am at my home in Hollywood, California, I climb 2,000-foot Mt. Hollywood and jog all the way down.

When I return home after exercising, then I am ready to have some kind of fresh fruit such as a papaya or pineapple for I have earned it. Then I settle down to my typewriter to answer my voluminous correspondence, to work on this book, or write an article for a health magazine.

The physical perfection and mental alertness of the Maori race, of whose natural diet I have already spoken, must also be attributed to their combination of proper nutrition with proper exercise.

Few primitive races have developed calisthenic and systematic physical exercise to so high a degree as the Maori. On arising early in the morning, the chief of the village starts singing a song accompanied by a rhythmic dance. This is taken up not only by the members of his household, but also by all the adjoining households, until the entire village is swaying in unison to the same tempo. This has a remarkably beneficial effect in developing deep breathing, as well as muscles of the body, particularly those of the abdomen . . . with the result that these people maintain excellent figures to the last day of their lives.

The Maori race developed a knowledge of nature's laws and adopted a system of living in harmony with those laws to so high a degree that they were able to build what early scientists reported as the most perfect race on the face of the earth.

A BIG BREAKFAST DOES NOT GIVE YOU ENERGY

There cannot be genuine hunger unless the food has been earned by physical activity. Furthermore, it is not true that a big breakfast gives you energy for the morning and the rest of the day.

When you eat a meal, it must be digested . . . and then by the process of metabolism broken down into waste matter, with the release of energy. This process is not accomplished by the body in minutes. It requires hours to thoroughly digest and metabolize one's food.

So, how is it possible to get quick energy and vitality out of a big breakfast? Instead of giving energy, it requires energy to digest and metabolize what you have eaten. If you are going to eat breakfast, you must earn it by several hours of strenuous physical activity.

With most people today, however, the reverse is the rule. They get out of bed, go to the bathroom, then sit down to a big breakfast. Have they earned it? The answer is absolutely, "No!"

When I see people stuffing heavy breakfasts into themselves, or into their families, I shudder to think of the brainwashing accomplished by the greedy, powerful commercial food industry. Housewives are constantly being told that growing children should be sent to school with the stomach filled with food. They hear how delicious this or that cereal is, how mouth-watering are Aunt Josie's pancakes, how luscious are so-and so's doughnuts . . . how wonderful Yoo-Yoo coffee is . . . how tasty ham and bacon are . . . how strengthening eggs are.

Homemakers hear this day in and day out on radio and TV, read it in their daily newspapers . . . and they start to believe that a big breakfast is necessary to health and strength, and what a pleasure it is to sit down to a big breakfast.

This type of brainwashing is increasing hedonism (the doctrine

74

that pleasure is the principle good) . . . and consumerism (to use up something whether you need it or not). This is the creed of the big commercial food producers.

The healthiest and most nutritious food for the morning is fresh fruit. It is easily digested, and it provides those vitamins, minerals and nutrients with which your body needs to be replenished.

My five children ate only fresh fruit for breakfast, and they could outrun and outclimb all their playmates and outshine every child in school work. Also, they were free from the miserable mucus which plagues most children who eat a big breakfast.

LET CHILDREN DEVELOP A HEALTHY HUNGER

My program of earning my breakfast by strenuous physical activity actually began in my childhood on a big farm in Virginia. From the time I can remember, I arose at 4 a.m. to do my share of the farm chores. My father first assigned me to feeding our hundreds of chickens. As I grew bigger and stronger I chopped kindling wood for the morning fires in the cookstove and fireplaces. (No central heating in those days.)

At seven years of age I was doing hard physical labor from 4 to 7 a.m., when breakfast was served. My family and all the hired hands were working hard during those same three hours, often in bitter cold weather trudging through knee-deep snow. When we reached the breakfast table we were hungry . . . a healthy hunger, because we had earned our food.

I receive many inquiries today from mothers who are distressed because their children refuse to eat healthful, nourishing food, but instead stuff themselves with commercial dead-food "junk".

Since even farms are highly mechanized today, and practically every household is equipped with labor saving gadgets, the healthy hunger developed by early morning chores is denied to modern youngsters. Instead, they watch early morning "children's programs" on TV, whose sponsors extol the delicious taste and body-building qualities of dead cereals, refined white sugar products, cakes and cookies made with refined white flour and hydrogenated shortening, cola and soft drinks, hot dogs,

75

hamburgers and pizza pies. So these children are brainwashed into wanting such foodless foods.

At the Health Resort which I operated for 25 years, I had a special department for such children. At first most of them turned up their noses at the salads, properly cooked vegetables, fresh fruit and nuts, and other natural foods.

So, I let them go hungry until they decided to eat what was put before them. Fasting on distilled water detoxifies a child's body as well as an adult's . . . and a child will become internally cleansed and develop a healthy hunger much more quickly than an adult.

Within one or two days, those children were so hungry that they were willing to eat anything I gave them! I fed them delicious, nutritious health meals . . . and explained to them why it is necessary to eat good, natural food. During the few days of fasting their perverted taste buds had returned to normal, and they soon developed a real, natural taste for wholesome health foods. Within a few weeks they would eat nothing else. Their taste buds as well as their bodies rejected the dead-foods.

If you have similar problems with your children, and are as desperate as some mothers who write me, let your children go hungry for a day or two. Confine them in an airy room with plenty of distilled water. It won't harm them . . . it will help them develop a healthy hunger which you can satisfy with healthy food. **Never make a compromise — make it natural foods or nothing!** You will be surprised how quickly and effectively this works. It may be harder for you to discipline yourself than to discipline your children . . . but stick to your guns, and you will both benefit.

12 MEALS WEEKLY

As stated at the beginning of this book, malnutrition among the overfed is as dangerous to health as malnutrition among the underfed. It is what you eat — not how much.

Like many health-minded people around the world, I find that I can keep in the pink of condition on 12 natural food meals a week. As previously noted, I fast one 24-hour period each week, and never eat breakfast. My morning snack, after three hours of outdoor exercise, is fresh fruit.

Around 1 p.m. I eat my first meal of the day. This usually begins with a large salad made of grated raw carrots, grated raw cabbage, grated raw beets, chopped celery, parsley, watercress, avocado, radishes, and other fresh raw vegetables that are available. I make my salad dressing of fresh lemon juice, (Patricia, my daughter, prefers fresh orange), pure apple cider vinegar and an unsaturated oil such as safflower, soy, peanut, corn or olive. (We add garlic to our dressing and kelp seasoning and other salad herbs.)

Then I have a cooked vegetable, usually a different one each day for variety. Here in Hawaii we can purchase fresh green soy beans, and a cooked dish of this nourishing food is among my favorites. There is always a variety of raw nuts and seeds, dates, figs and raisins on the table.

I believe in spacing one's meals far apart, so when you come to the table you have a natural hunger, not merely an appetite. So my second meal of the day is around 7 p.m. I start this evening meal with another kind of salad such as cole slaw or lettuce with tomatoes, cucumbers and avocado. I try to eat an avocado every day.

After the salad, another freshly cooked vegetable . . . and several times weekly a baked white potato, yam or sweet potato. Now, if my body tells me I need a piece of fish or meat or an egg, I eat it.

My diet is mixed, although most of my eating is vegetarian. It is a satisfying diet for me, and since I happen to be a very good cook and know how to use herbs, my food is delicious as well as nutritious. (**There are more than 1,000 natural food recipes in my "Four Generation Health Food Cook Book".**) In shopping for food, I look for healthful variety.

I drink no liquids with my meals. Since I do not use salt or salty foods, I have no thirst at mealtime. My diet contains plenty of bulk, moisture and lubrication. I am never constipated. My bowels move on arising and again within an hour after eating . . . outgo should equal intake. I never have any gas, bloat or "stomach distress" of any kind. My entire digestive system from my mouth to my anus, a 30-foot span, works perfectly.

My liquid intake consists of fruit and vegetable juices and

distilled water, which I drink between meals. My only between-meal snacks consist of juicy fresh fruit — such as a cool slice of watermelon — or a glass of fresh fruit or vegetable juice.

At night before retiring I enjoy a warm cup of California Mint Tea, or some other natural herb tea.

Through my program of diet and exercise, I enjoy a superior state of bodily and mental health. My body and I are in harmony. We work together as a team. We have perfect communication.

DIETING WHILE TRAVELING

When traveling for business or pleasure, eating in restaurants presents many problems. I have solved this confusion by carrying a small "health tote bag" with nuts, seeds, dates, raisins, herbs, garlic, and the fresh fruit and vegetables that I purchase daily along the way.

My daughter Patricia and I have made seven trips around the world. In order to follow our system of diet, we have dubbed ourselves **"the best bathroom chefs in the world."** We carry a few stainless steel pans, a small chopping board, knives, small nut grinder, and a small one-plate electric burner. With this simple equipment we can prepare healthful, nourishing and delicious meals anywhere!

We enjoy going to the large farmers markets in different parts of the world and selecting our own food. In many foreign countries organically grown foods are fortunately the only kind they can afford to raise. A compost pile costs the small farmer nothing. He does not have the money for commercial fertilizers and pesticides.

The food in these markets is always fresh. The small farmers bring it in and dispose of it in a few hours. And there is such a variety of foods to choose from.

If you eat fish, the fish were caught the night before. All the meat, chickens, lamb have been freshly slaughtered.

One of my favorite markets is in Tahiti. The market opens promptly at 5 a.m. and closes at 7 a.m. Here you can purchase an array of freshly picked tropical fruits such as papaya, mangos, bananas, pineapples and many other delicious fruits. There are fresh, organically grown vegetables . . . and many, many other kinds of fresh foods. And of course, the fresher the foods, the more nutrients they contain.

A basic rule for healthful nutrition while traveling is to simplify your eating. Patricia and I have learned from long experience "on the road" that the simpler you eat, the healthier you are and the more endurance and energy you have!

Many times during our travels we live on a mono-diet . . . that is, eating just one item at a meal. At one meal we will have all fruit . . . at another, we will have a nourishing soup made of vegetables, lentils, or leeks and potatoes. Many times we make an entire meal on a large avocado salad.

Of course, we could indulge in a 12-course meal at a restaurant or hotel . . . but then we would have to eat salted food and a meal composed of too many mixtures.

Too much food encourages overeating. You should get up from every meal feeling that you could have eaten just a little more — and that rule holds, whether traveling or not!

NATURAL FOODS ARE MEDICINES

Wherever you go, you will sooner or later encounter amateur or professional "diet experts" who are prejudiced against one or more of the natural foods. In every such case which I have investigated — and there have been many — the prejudice has been based not upon factual data, but upon a purely personal reaction.

For example, I knew a nutritionist who had a delicate, weak stomach and intestinal tract. He suffered from mucus colitis, and could not tolerate coarse, raw foods such as carrots, beets, cabbage, celery, radishes, etc. So he wrote a book condemning all coarse foods and advocating a bland diet for everyone.

Another claimed that fresh cherries should not be eaten, as this fruit was harmful to the liver and gall bladder. The only research he had done was on himself. Cherries did not agree with him . . . therefore, no one should eat cherries. Probably the reason that cherries disagreed with him was because he also drank coffee with cream and refined white sugar, or chocolate or some other devitalized food, and the fresh cherries were acting as a detoxifying agent to cleanse his liver and gall bladder of toxic poisons.

Remember, as Hippocrates said . . .

"Natural foods are medicines."

All human bodies carry toxic poisons. When natural foods enter the system they start to clean house . . . and, as explained previously, this usually causes temporary discomfort. The degree and duration of the discomfort depends upon the amount of toxic poisons stored within the body.

When I was a boy on a Virginia farm I ate a one-sided, devitalized diet. Whenever I ate strawberries I broke out with big, swollen hives. I told everyone that strawberries were unfit to eat because they gave me hives. I did not realize that the strawberries were detoxifying my body. Today, with a relatively toxic free body, I can eat all the strawberries I desire without getting hives.

When some nutritionist tells you not to eat a certain food, find out how much factual, documentary evidence he has to support his claims.

NUTRITION IS A YOUNG SCIENCE

Remember that nutritional science is very young. More research must be done to clarify the confusion which is cluttering up this science today. All kinds of people, some qualified and many totally unqualified, are teaching nutrition. In deciding on your own program of eating, be guided by documented facts and your own intelligence.

Man has survived on this earth for a long, long time on many different diets. There are all sorts of people in the world today eating all sorts of foods and living long, healthy lives.

"Put a knife to thy throat, if thou be a man given to appetite."
— Solomon

Life cannot be maintained unless life be taken in, and this is best done by making at least 60 percent of your diet raw and cooked vegetables, with a plentiful supply of fresh juicy fruits.
— Patricia Bragg

Jesus said: "Thy faith hath made thee whole, and go and sin no more." and that means your dietetic sins. He himself, through fasting and prayer, was able to heal the sick and cure all manner of diseases.

One point on which unbiased, qualified nutritionists whole heartedly agree is that the modern devitalized foods are the basic cause of all the nutritional problems of our civilization.

It is time for the science of nutrition to be researched and taught on a mature, intelligent basis. All people interested in superior health want all the facts they can get on balanced, healthful nutrition.

YOU AND YOUR DIET

We all know that the greatest step in the improvement of our nutrition is completely discarding devitalized foods. We all agree that raw and properly cooked fruits and vegetables are very important to good nutrition.

Now from this point on, each person must build his diet with the natural foods best suited for his body chemistry.

If the fruitarian diet appeals to you, by all means give it a trial.

If the fruit and nut diet sounds logical to you, try it.

If the fruit and meat diet appeals to you, experiment with it and find out if it's for you.

If the strict all raw food diet appeals to you, give it a trial.

And so with the exclusively vegetarian or lacto-vegetarian diet. You are the important person when it comes to selecting a diet for yourself.

We know that the mixed diet — combining raw and cooked fruits and vegetables, meat, fish, poultry, whole grains, eggs, nuts, seeds, dairy products such as milk, cheese and yogurt — has the greatest appeal to the greatest number seeking good nutrition.

Select or experiment with the various diets until you find the one that you feel is going to do the most good for you. Only you know how you feel, how much physical and mental energy you have, and how you look. In selecting a diet take all these factors into consideration.

And always reserve the right to change your mind — and your diet — any time.

This is intelligent selection of a good, healthful diet . . . and I assure you, you will no longer be confused by the diet experts or anyone else who talks nutrition to you.

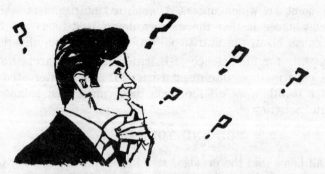

TYPICAL QUESTIONS FROM THE CONFUSED

Here are samplings from my mail and lecture audiences, which cover some of the most frequently asked questions by nutrition-confused people.

QUESTION:

I read in a health book that you should never mix fruit and vegetables at the same meal. The article went on to say that fruit and vegetables at the same meal were absolutely incompatible and could only bring on malnutrition and cell starvation. The two, when they were mixed, would cause gas bloat and could lead to serious troubles of the digestive tract. What is you opinion of this statement?

ANSWER:

Prof. Arnold Ehret, who in my personal opinion was one of the greatest nutritionists of our times, had this to say about fruit and vegetables.

My experience has taught me that only raw celery, lettuce, carrots and beets combine well with fruits. In general, it is best never to use more than three kinds with the same combination. Always use one kind as the prevailing stock or base. For a bad, acid or mucused stomach use menus consisting of more vegetables and little fruits. For a stomach in better condition, or average stomach, use more fruits and less vegetables."

Again in his book he makes this important statement: "Always eat fruit first. The digestion of ripe fruits takes place

82

within a normal stomach within a few minutes after eating. Wait five to ten minutes before eating a vegetable course."

In France it is the custom to serve a large basket of many kinds of fresh fruit at the end of every meal. My mother was French and she carried out this custom all of her long healthy life. The Hawaiians — one of the healthiest races of people on earth, until the white man started his complete degeneration with dead-devitalized food — ate fruit and vegetables together. At their luaus (feast of Hawaiian food) they serve an abundance of fruit and vegetables to visitors to the islands today. I know many healthy Hawaiians who mix fruit and vegetables with every meal they eat.

However, you must be the final judge whether you are going to eat fruit and vegetables at the same meal. No one can feel what goes on in your digestive tract but you yourself. Personally, I like the Ehret plan of eating fruit at the first part of the meal. On some occasions, after eating a meal of raw salad and cooked vegetables, I enjoy some kind of fresh fruit. I have never had any kind of unpleasant reaction from this combination. My experimental animals from the jungles, such as the chimpanzee and baboon, enjoyed fruit and vegetables at the same meal. They are natural and healthy vegetarians.

Both fruit and vegetables are the most natural foods one can eat, and it is beyond my logic and reason not to mix them at the same meal.

QUESTION:

I read an article in a well-known health magazine titled **"The Harder the Water the Safer the Heart".** It states that it's calcium carbonate that makes water hard, and calcium that is essential to heart health. It went on to say that scientific studies have established that when drinking water which is soft, there is a marked tendency towards increased deficiencies in tooth and bone formation and increased tooth decay. Of course, they are talking about water softener chemical equipment on both the hot and cold faucets. Please give your opinion on this subject.

ANSWER:

I would under no circumstances drink water that is softened by a chemical household water softener. The sodium content of artificially softened water is high (sodium is not used in healthful diets), and very undesirable and dangerous to many cases of heart trouble. Sodium collects in the body, attracts water to itself and brings overweight or edema (swelling), both of which increase the work of an already overworked heart.

I am a biochemist with more than 60 years of continuous practice and research, and it is very difficult for me to understand how people can make the statement that inorganic calcium carbonate found in hard water is good for the heart and the body.

In the desert town in California where I have a home, the mineral drinking water is highly saturated with inorganic calcium carbonate and many other inorganic minerals. I have lived in this mineral water area for many years, and I find that people who drink this hard mineral water die long before their time, many of them with heart problems and hardening of the arteries. There is a great amount of arthritis, kidney stones, gall stones, and bladder stones among the townspeople who drink this highly saturated inorganic mineral water. They all seem to walk as though their spines and joints are cemented. There are plenty of prematurely aged people here.

I seem to be the only person in the higher age bracket who jogs every day, climbs the mountains which surround this town and takes long swims in the spa pools. I drink only steam processed distilled water. I get my calcium as well as the other organic minerals from the fruits, vegetables, and food I eat, and by taking my organic minerals in natural food supplements.

I would personally like to invite all the doctors and chemists who make such statements that water with many natural (inorganic) minerals is the best for drinking to come here and live and drink this highly inorganic mineralized water. I know it would not be long before our local undertaker would be doing a rush business on these people.

QUESTION:
Why do health magazines, some health lecturers and health food stores try and get people to take Dolomite tablets, which are supposed to be rich in magnesium and calcium? They must know these are made of powdered inorganic limestone that has been ground to extra fineness and then baked. They

84

claim easy assimilation. Easy assimilation to where in the human body? Maybe in the arteries causing hardening of the arteries, or in the kidneys to form kidney stones, gall stones or bladder stones, or maybe arthritis of the spine and joints of the body.

I was a chemistry major at my university and taught chemistry in a college for four years before my marriage. As a chemist I definitely know the difference between an organic and an inorganic mineral. I know the human body can only assimilate an organic mineral. When will people wake up to chemical science?

ANSWER:

Don't blame the health food stores for carrying Dolomite. They are in business to serve health-minded people what they demand. If the customers have been brainwashed by health magazines and health lecturers that Dolomite is rich in magnesium and calcium and should be taken as a regular food supplement, their business is to give the customers what they demand.

There are hundreds of products in the modern health food store. Many health food store owners personally do not approve of some of these items, but their customers demand them and there is nothing a store owner can do but serve them. I have a personal friend who owns a large health food store. She is a strict raw fooder. But her business is to serve the health-minded persons what they want, not what she wants.

I have some encouraging news for you, however. Several years ago when the Dolomite craze hit the health food minded, most every manufacturer of food supplements produced a Dolomite and spent large sums advertising and promoting it. But today it is a dying duck. Very few food supplement manufacterers produce Dolomite anymore. It is rapidly dying on the vine. In another year I do not believe you will be able to purchase the stuff. The health-minded people are getting smarter every day.

QUESTION:

My father has cancer of the prostate gland. My aunt has put him on a natural diet for the past two years and he seems to get no worse and goes about his daily tasks. He has no pain or distress. My uncle, who has just returned from California, brought back some Desert Indian herb tea and assures my father that if he will faithfully drink this tea he will be cured. **What is your opinion of Desert Indian tea?**

ANSWER:

First, let me definitely state that I certainly wish Desert Indian herb tea were a certain cure of cancer. It would truly be a godsend to all the poor humans who have cancer. I know your uncle has good intentions towards your father.

Twenty-five hundred years ago on the island of Cos in Greece a teacher-physician, Hippocrates, told his assembled natural healing students in one of his profound statements, **"Your food will be your medicine and your medicine will be your food."** No one in these many years has more eloquently given us the truth about the power of food being a healer. Look at Vitamin C — it's a cure for scurvy, and B-Complex is a cure for beri-beri. Indians and other primitive people have found remarkable cures with plants and herbs. But at this present moment we know little about the healing powers of Desert Indian tea. The Desert Indians have been using it for centuries for all kinds of physical problems. But there is no recorded factual, documented evidence that Desert Indian tea is a cure for cancer. Therefore, it is my personal opinion that until qualified scientists have made a most thorough investigation of the merits of this tea, I believe your uncle is giving your father false hope. By all means, have your father drink Desert Indian tea. Nothing but a trial beats a failure. But explain to him that to date there has been no cure-all for cancer. Keep him on a natural food program.

QUESTION:

I have arthritis in practically all the joints of my body. This has been going on for ten years. I read health magazines and books and follow a good clean wholesome diet. I have never taken any kind of medication or pain killers. I take hot mineral baths, exercise, massage and light therapy. Even though it is painful I take long walks and exercise the best my joints will take. With this program the arthritis has been held under control.

My very good neighbor who is health minded made me a present of several pounds of alfalfa seeds, and told me to make a tea and that it would cure my arthritis. She is so enthusaistic about this tea. Naturally, I am like a drowning person grasping for a straw. **What do you know about alfalfa seed tea as a cure for arthritis?**

ANSWER:

I wish with all my heart that alfalfa seed tea was an absolute, definite cure for arthritis, as we have over 20 million Americans suffering from this misery. Like Desert Indian tea as a cure for cancer, there is no recorded documented evidence that alfalfa seed tea will cure arthritis. I have heard diet specialists say there was, but I knew they were giving false hope to suffering humans. I am very skeptical about the word "cure". Curing is done by the basic biological functions of the body. Ever since man began to have diseases he has been looking for cures. In the first records of healing, written in Egyptian hieroglyphics thousands of years before the Christian era, are inscribed magic food formulas for curing disease. Even in those days, man wanted cures for his miseries. In short, he thought in terms of magic — a magic that never was, a magic that never will be.

Find a good natural eating program for yourself, and there may be that "magic" healing power in it for your problem. It takes not just one food to work magic in your body — it takes a rounded out, balanced, cleansing diet and fasting to regain and maintain health. Read, study, and never get confused. Live close to Nature and listen to what Nature tells you to do.

QUESTION:

Practically all diet experts advise mothers to load their children with milk. I am confused. **Is it possible for a child to drink too much milk?**

ANSWER:

Yes, if milk is consumed in such large amounts that it crowds out other important foods from the diet. (I discussed milk more thoroughly in another section of this book.)

QUESTION:

My son is 23 years of age and is 5 feet 6 inches in height, and until his illness he weighed 190 pounds. **He is a weight lifter and often exercises three or four hours at a time.** The magazines he reads show the big muscle men with great body bulk. The diet experts who publish these magazines tell the boys to bulk-up, eat protein pills by the handfulls, drink rich protein drinks, eat large amounts of meat, eggs, cheese and drink gallons of milk. **I have been telling my son that muscle overweight is bad as fat, and that too much body bulk puts an extra strain on the heart.** With all my son's big muscles, with all his strength, five weeks ago he came down with double pneumonia, and for two weeks in the hospital's intensive care ward he hovered between life and death. Just two weeks before this happened he won two award cups for his powerful and beautiful muscular body. In the five weeks in the hospital he has lost much of this bulk. You have been an athlete, please help me help my son find the true way to a healthy life.

ANSWER:

Big, powerful, bulging muscles do not necessarily mean internal health! There is a vast difference between perfect health and mere physical fitness. Your son was physically fit, but he was far from being healthy.

Athletes who are only physically fit live no longer than the average person who never exercises. Sandow, the greatest strong man who ever lived, died of a stroke at the age of 58. Bill Tilden, the greatest tennis player of this century, died at 57 of a heart attack.

I have been an athlete for many, many years, but I believe in nutritional fitness as well as physical fitness. I do not approve of bulking-up the human body with enormous amounts of protein. This is not a balanced diet.

When I was in active practice as a Naturopathic doctor, my office was filled with athletes and others who were suffering from the results of a prolonged high protein diet. Protein foods contain plenty of uric acid . . . and the uncontrolled intake of uric acid can produce an imbalance in the body chemistry which results in many miseries. The most frequent and painful of these miseries is arthritic gout.

Many of the diet experts who preach the high protein diet theory have a money-getting motivation behind their advice. You will usually find that they have protein pills and protein drinks to sell.

Of course, the more calories one eats, the bigger he is prone to get. These human derricks may look good, but it is all for show. One's weight must be normal to one's structure and body frame to be both physically fit and nutritionally healthy.

I have buried all the big-muscle boys who were in their athletic prime with me. I have a good, normal body for sports. I am a jogger, a swimmer, a mountain climber, a tennis player. I enjoy my barbells and dumbell exercises, but I use these weights only to firm and tone my muscles. My height is 5 feet, 8 inches, and I have maintained my weight at 150 to 155 pounds for a long time. I accomplish this by the balanced combination of a physical fitness program with proper nutrition.

The thousands who exercise daily with barbells, yoga, track and field sports, gymnastic equipment, with pick and shovel, plow and pitchfork — but neglect healthful nutrition — have no desirable record of longevity. Lengthening human life is primarily a matter of preventing disease. The principle causes of death after middle-life are heart disease, cancer, kidney disease, pneumonia and kindred degenerative diseases. We must fight off these killers with a pure, clean bloodstream that is built from the foods we eat and the liquids we drink.

The first exercise is a mental one. We must learn to discipline ourselves. We must learn not to overeat, even on good natural foods. We must learn to push away from the dinner table feeling that we could eat just a little more. We must eat a balanced, natural diet.

Our great enemy is toxic poison. This is the killer we must fight, and it can only be done with nutritional knowledge. Some physical fitness experts will tell you that exercise will burn up all toxic poisons. That is true to a certain extent, but it will not burn them all up. Toxic poisons are disease breeders. We can help keep disease out of our bodies by a combination of proper nutrition and a program of physical fitness personally suited to our own body.

Select the kind of exercise that you enjoy doing . . . that gives you mental relaxation as well as muscular and circulatory stimulation. You want to feel a carefree lightness to your body . . . to create a feeling of agelessness . . . to feel the joy of effort.

Let me say again that, contrary to popular opinion, an athletic physique is by no means an indication of perfect internal health. Unnumbered thousands of people have suffered quite long enough under the great delusion that longevity and superior internal health are associated in some mysterious way with physical development. Let's be done, once and for all, with this fallacy.

When your son comes home from the hospital, try to show him the folly of trying to be an over-sized monster. Maybe this battle with death will put reason and logic into your son's mind. He can enjoy his weight training and still have a clean-cut moderately-built athletic body. But he must never get back to bulking his body with a high protein diet. It's a lean horse for a long race.

QUESTION:

My sister has had a serious weight problem for many years. Every crash diet that some diet expert writes about, she goes into it heart and soul. I know of at least 20 crash diets she has followed. Her latest reducing fad is with a group of other overweight women. They meet and openly discuss their overweight problem which is good. But she gets a magazine from this organization with menus and recipes that are atrocious — the dead devitalized foods they put together is unbelievable. They deal exclusively in calories. If the recipe is low in calories they can put any kind of "trash" in their bodies. There is absolutely no nutritional balance, no thought of vitamins, minerals, enzymes and natural nutrients. My sister as a consequence has lost weight, but she also has lost much of her good health. She is tired all the time. Her skin and muscle tone are bad. She is ashen gray and has big dark circles under her eyes and her eyes look lifeless. I don't believe that the diet experts behind these weight reducing organizations have had any scientific training in nutrition. This is very confusing to me as I love my sister and do not like her to be in this wretched physical condition. What would you suggest?

ANSWER:

You are so right about many of the reducing diet experts. At calorie counting they are fine, but nutritionally ignorant! The very best suggestion I can give you is to sit down with your sister and tell her that although she is reducing, at the same time she is damaging her health by incorrect eating. Explain to her that she can build a healthy diet from natural foods with a low calorie count and lose weight and gain health at the same time. May I suggest you give her my book, **"How To Reduce**

Nature's Way". I think this may be the answer to her problem. I have helped thousands of people reduce without endangering their health or their personal appearance.

QUESTION:

I just purchased a new book on Nutrition and Health. **The author writes about raw fruit and vegetable juice with the following advice:** For anemia take equal portions of beet, celery and parsley juice; for bronchitis take carrot and garlic in equal parts; for diabetes take carrot, spinach and dandelion juice. For gall stones take celery and parsley juice. Then she writes about certain foods: brazil nuts good for greater sexual activity; cashew nuts good for low vitality; blackberry leaves bruised and applied outwardly help heal piles; raspberries remove cankers from mucous membrane, good for dysentery; brussel sprouts good for eyesight and skin; okra for stomach ulcers; onions are an anti-bacterial infection fighter — sauteed in butter they will neutralize the urine in diabetic patients; pumpkin good for weak eyes, nose and throat. And many, many other cures with certain foods. What is your opinion about these so-called cures?

ANSWER:

As a nutritionist and biochemist for 60 years, I wish the curing of these ailments were that easy. I think many sick people who adopt these suggestions are going to be greatly disappointed. Defeating a long standing ailment is something more than a few juice combinations and certain foods. First, a person must stop all eating and drinking of devitalized materials. Then there must be a period of fasting to detoxify the body. There must be a balanced nutritional diet for cleansing the body of toxic poisons, toxic mucus derived from undigested and uneliminated, unnatural food substances, which has been accumulating in the body for years. People want symptoms relieved. They do not want to find the cause of their ailments. They want a magic cure. Disease is an effort of the body to rid itself of toxic poison, toxic mucus and other vicious toxemias, and my naturopathic methods assist nature in purifying the body. Not the symptom but the entire body is to be healed; it must be thoroughly cleansed, absolutely freed from long standing toxic poison. My method is not a cure . . . it is a regeneration, by body detoxification and ridding the body of putrid material it has accumulated since childhood.

Your body must have a thorough housecleaning. When the cleansing is accomplished, you will have superior purified, splendid health such as you never knew before.

During the time you are undergoing the toxic housecleaning, there will be periods in which you will experience the "healing crisis" . . . you will be feeling miserable, for at that time you will be loosening and eliminating body toxins. It takes from one to four years to bring the body to a perfect state of ageless health. Most people do not have the patience and the intestinal fortitude to go through a detoxification period. They want the easy magic cure. If their sexual power fades, they will be glad to regain it by eating brazil nuts.

I toiled for 60 years as a Naturopathic doctor using the natural sciences to aid sick people to find superior health. There are no easy roads to curing a disease. That is the reason mankind sickens and dies long before his time . . . that is why hospitals and mental institutions are filled to overflowing with the diseased and the hopeless. Certainly people will purchase Health Books that offer a "quick cure" with juices or food. I read the health magazines and books and I am amazed at the "sure cures" people can get with this food or that food.

It takes years of pains-taking research work for the sound evaluation of a cure by a certain food. It took years and years to prove that Vitamin C was a cure for scurvy. Unhappily, sick people consider health something they can find by eating this special food or combination of juices or something they can purchase in a bottle. They forget, or never knew, that superior health can only be gained by strictly obeying the basic laws of nature.

Hippocrates' great precept was that Nature is the only healer. He was Nature's assistant by giving the sick natural foods that purify the body, plenty of oxygen, exercise, sound sleep, recreation, fasting, and rest from pressures.

My books, **"The Miracle of Fasting"** and **"The Toxicless Diet and Healing System"**, will show you that the prevention, elimination and management of disease may be gained without special so-called "cures". Your body is self-cleansing (if you will give it a chance) self-repairing and self-healing.

Yes, the "quick cure" books are flooding the book shops and

there are many more to come. Shakespeare said, "What fools we mortals be." And there is an old German saying, "Even the gods stand helpless before stupidity." And the world's great showman P.T. Barnum said, "There is a sucker born every minute."

Many sick humans reaching out for health are prone to be gullible and easily duped when it comes to fast and easy cures.

Health is Wealth and it must be earned.

QUESTION:

At our nutritional club a speaker told us that we should not drink the juices of fruit and vegetables. In fact, he stated that we should not even drink any kind of water, not even distilled. He stated that by eating an abundance of raw whole fruit and vegetables and waterless cooked vegetables, we would supply our bodies with plenty of liquid; and that if we drank fruit and vegetable juices and water, these would only overwork and burden our kidneys.

I have been drinking fruit and vegetable juices and distilled water for years, and have superior health. I have never had a trace of kidney distress.

What is your opinion of this speaker's theory?

ANSWER:

I speak to many sincere nutritional clubs around the world. People who belong to these groups are the sincere health students seeking knowledge and wisdom on good nutrition and health habits. But at meeting after meeting, one speaker after the other comes out with some theories on eating which, in my opinion, are only confusing to these health seekers.

The preponderance of evidence is that a moderate amount of raw fruit and vegetable juices are healthful, and that distilled water is the only water fit to enter the human body. Distilled water is pure H_2O, free from all inorganic minerals that do great damage to the body.

I would demand from any speaker who condemns an established nutritional pattern to furnish documentary evidence that his theory has had qualified investigation by graduate biochemists whose specialty is nutritional research.

There are many, many speakers lecturing before nutritional groups who are giving their personal opinions on nutrition rather

93

than documented factual evidence. And that is one of the reasons we have so very much confusion in the field of nutrition. Have these speakers qualified themselves to be authorities on nutrition? Are they graduate biochemists? Can they go into a nutritional laboratory and prove conclusively what they say? Have they made test feedings on laboratory animals and humans? Do they have the research to prove and qualify their statements?

Don't let any speaker confuse you. Ask him to give you factual evidence on his theory. If he can produce such evidence, then you can make your decision to accept or reject the theory.

Qualified scientists do not deal in their opinions, but in facts, which can be proven over and over again to any biochemist.

So continue, as I do, to drink raw fruit and vegetable juices in moderation as well as distilled water and have no fears that your kidneys are going to fail you. Or, if you wish, try this speaker's theory and see what happens. You must be the final judge of what goes into your body.

QUESTION:

I suffer with attacks of the gout. Every doctor tells me something different to eat. At last I found a nutritionist who told me to drink cherry juice from the health food store and eat canned or fresh unsweetened sour Ann cherries along with a strictly vegetarian diet. It was the first common sense information that appealed to my intelligence. The others only confused me. What is your opinion of this type of diet for combating gout?

ANSWER:

I will go along 100% with the diet information this nutritionist has given you. But I want you to remember cherries are not a cure for gout. They do, however, have a way, along with a vegetarian diet, of lowering the uric acid level in the blood. Uric acid is the villain that makes gout a painful misery. Along with this diet I suggest that you fast one 24-hour period a week. And three or four times a year take a fast of from 7 to 10 days, and really get that uric acid down to a normal level. My book, **"The Miracle of Fasting"**, should be your nutritional Bible to help guide you to perfect health.

QUESTION:

My ten-year-old son suffers from terrible attacks of asthma.

I have taken him to three well-known nutritionists, and two of them tell me to let the boy drink plenty of milk, but one said to drink it only in moderation. I have been reading some of your books, and you state that a child suffering from asthma or bronchitis should never drink milk. Now, as a result, you nutritionists have me in a state of utter confusion and bewilderment. My boy is really suffering and I do not know which way to turn to help him.

ANSWER:

You are so very right, and you have a perfect right to be boiling mad because the nutritionists can really confuse the people.

But let's look on the other side of the coin. If your boy drinks milk and continues to have asthma attacks, does that not prove to you that commercial milk is mucus forming and that your boy should not have it?

If you have thoroughly read some of my books, you know definitely I am not for children drinking commercial milk of any kind after they have been weaned. And if the mother does not breast feed her child, goat's milk is superior to cow's milk.

Parents give milk to children because of its calcium content. Let me tell you there are many other foods free from mucus that have a high calcium content. A mixture of blanched almonds and soy powder along with orange juice in the blender makes a milk substitute . . . to this can be added brewers yeast and a teaspoon of black strap molasses.

The milk industry has so brainwashed the mothers of America about the importance of milk that they have become slaves to its use. I reared five healthy, husky, vigorous, strong children without the use of milk. Cows today are sick, kept in barns and are given all kinds of heavy medicines. Milk to me is bacteriological soup. It is the perfect food for breeding any germ, bug or virus.

Now it is up to you to make the decision; shall you or shall you not give milk to your boy suffering with asthma?

QUESTION:

At a P.T.A. meeting a doctor told our group that mothers worried too much about what they should feed their children, and that a child pretty much could decide what it wanted to eat.

I have three children and all they want to eat is what you call "trash food". When they go shopping for food with me they want hot dogs, white buns, cola drinks, dry commercial cereals, cookies, cakes, candies, canned soups, cans of pork and beans, chili, spaghetti, and nothing of nutritional value. What is a mother to do?

ANSWER:

In my personal opinion, I do not believe a child can select its own food. Many children do select their own foods . . . and as a result, this country is full of half-sick and very sick children.

You are the only one — if you have read and studied natural nutrition — to select and prepare natural foods for your children. They are not qualified in any way to select a well-balanced diet for themselves.

Do the greater part of your food shopping in a health food store. Keep the "trash foods" out of your kitchen. And don't make compromises with your children. That means no snacking of ice cream candy, cake, potato chips, french fried potatoes, greasy fried chicken, cremated hamburgers.

Sit down and explain to your children why you are feeding them health foods. Telling them merely that these are "good for them" is a total waste of time. You must communicate with your children, so that they understand why you feed them natural foods. Tell them you want them to be strong and healthy, to have teeth free from decay and a body free from colds and sickness. If you do not capture their interest and their minds in behalf of good nutrition, the great "trash food" industry will.

Good nutriton is first on the list for building healthy, mentally balanced children.

While on a hike in Hawaii a few weeks ago I came upon a group of youngsters in their early teens who were smoking "pot" (marijuana). I got into a friendly conversation with them and in the course of this conversation I asked about the kind of food they ate and every one of the twelve except one had been reared on "trash foods". The one who was not smoking marijuana was the one who told me that he was brought up on health foods and still ate them. He said that he did not need "pot" to put him on a "trip" . . . he said he was always enjoying life. He then told me he was with this group to tell them the terrible dangers of using dope of any kind.

After some time with the "Pot" group the young man and I hiked back to the city. On the way he told me that he believed that kids reared on poor nutrition were the ones who were easy victims of dope. He told me that just before I came upon the group, he had been telling the kids the way to get rid of the craving for dope and stimulants was to go 100% on natural health foods. This boy was only seventeen years old but he had a mature and good mind. He belonged to a group in Hawaii who was trying to get the kids off the dope and he said the first step was to get on natural foods. Later he introduced me to many teenagers who had been saved from "pot" by natural foods. So, to save yourself many heartaches and sadness get your kids off "trash foods."

QUESTION:

I had a consultation with one of the greatest authorities in nutrition a few days ago and he told me that I must never under any circumstances eat the skin of potatoes as there are too many poisons in the skin. I reared my family of six children on scrubbed, tubbed and washed potatoes both baked and steamed. I insisted that the family eat the skins, as I had learned from other nutritionists that it was in the skin of the potato we would find the greater amount of nutrients. Now I am really confused about eating the skin of a potato. Help me, please.

ANSWER:

Like yourself, I reared my family on baked potatoes eating the skins. And I shall continue eating the skins of potatoes until I have the factual evidence to convince me I should not eat them.

Medium sized potatoes contain 7.7 grams of protein, .4 grams of fat, 62.8 grams of carbohydrates (which makes the potato basically a starch food), 26 milligrams of calcium, 195 milligrams of phosphorus, 2.3 milligrams of iron, 11 milligrams of sodium, 1,495 milligrams of potassium, a trace of Vitamin A, .39 milligrams of thiamine, .14 milligrams of riboflavin, 5.4 milligrams of niacin, 73 milligrams of ascorbic acid (Vitamin C). This analysis is taken from the agriculture research service of the U.S. Dept. of Agriculture.

Arnold Ehret has this to say about potatoes: "Potatoes are a little better than grain products because they contain more organic minerals and they do not make a sticky paste in the intestines." He advised eating the whole baked potato skin and all.

One of the most vigorous races of people I have ever met are the Irish, who live in the extreme northern part of Ireland. Their basic diet is potatoes and fish. They have no cancer or any other degenerative diseases and are the most rugged people I have ever met. They always eat the skin of their potatoes.

Alfred McCann, a great nutritionist, advised the drinking of potato skin broth several times weekly to get minerals into the body. His recipe was to scrub three or four potatoes and peel them, leaving about 1/4 inch of the inside of the potato with the skin. This was steamed in three cups of distilled water for 30 minutes and then served. He gave substantial documentary evidence that this was a great food tonic to the system. His theory was that sick people should be given this food tonic to help with their recovery. He advised this as the nutritional treatment for scurvy.

However, the commercial potato we eat today and the potato people ate 50 years ago are vastly different. Today's commercial potato has been grown in chemicalized commercial fertilizers and heavily sprayed with all kinds of poisonous insecticides to kill the persistant potato bug. Naturally some of these poisons are going to get into the potato itself as well as the skin. This is a chance we have to take when it is impossible to get organically grown potatoes. After all, we do live in a poisoned world.

Please ask the nutritionist whom you consulted to give you documentary evidence as to just what poisons are in the skin of the potato that makes it unfit to eat. Please send me a copy of his reply, and I will investigate. In the meantime, I suggest that you continue to eat the skin of the potato.

QUESTION:

I heard you lecture in Pittsburgh thirty years ago and have been a faithful follower of your teachings, but I am confused and must seek your assistance in my problem.

My husband and my two teenage sons are strictly meat, potato, apple pie and coffee men. My husband is far from being a well man but he passes off his aches and pains by saying, "It's just old age creeping up on me and you can not do anything about it".

A nutritional doctor, who is the head of the nutritional department of a large eastern university, has a column in one of our daily papers. No matter what you, Hauser, and the other natural nutritionists say or write, this man calls it "nutritional nonsense". He says that we are the best fed nation in the world, and that white bread, white sugar, white rice, salt, hot dogs, ham, processed cheese, dry commercial cereals, luncheon meats, ice cream, sprayed fruit and vegetables, cake mixes, canned soups, canned foods are good foods.

My family read these articles to me and ridicule my health food eating. In spite of my family's ridicule I continue to eat my health foods, because I have perfect health and am never ever sick. But this nagging does get frustrating sometimes.

ANSWER:

You have the courage of your convictions, so stand your ground. You have personally experienced the benefits of eating health foods. It is too bad that your sick, ailing husband and sons cannot see that you have proven by precept and example that health foods have given you good sound health.

I know of the newspaper writing nutritionist to whom you refer. He is supported by the 20 billion dollar food industry who continue trying to brainwash the American people into believing that our modern manufactured food is good food.

But the walls of these massive food industries are slowly crumbling. Men like Ralph Nader are exposing these giant food manufacturers. The first wall to come crumbling down on their heads was their $400 million a year dry cereal hoax. Congress investigated the dry cereal racket and found there was more nourishment in the paper boxes which contained the "empty calorie" dry cereal.

And the very man you are writing about is on the payroll of one, if not the largest, of these dry cereal manufacturers. So his word means absolutely nothing when he writes about today's "trashy" dead, devitalized foods.

Too bad about your family, they are on their way to the Sick and Die Clinic.

QUESTION:

At our P.T.A. meeting the other night a well-known doctor spoke on nutrition. He stated that canned fruit and vegetable juices found in the grocery stores were just as nutritious as freshly made juices. He stated that the sprays on our fruits and vegetables were so low that they could not possibly hurt us. He stated that pasteurized milk was far superior to raw milk and he said that organic fertile eggs were no better than ordinary eggs. He ridiculed wheat germ, brewers yeast, honey, whole grain foods and cereals and health food in general, called them "faddist foods". He said that the only one who profited when health foods were purchased was the store owner.

But here is where I got my laughs on this so-called authority. He was at least 30 pounds overweight, had false teeth that clattered when he talked, thick bifocal glasses, and a hearing aid stuck in his ear — and on top of that he was sniffling all evening.

And yet my husband and daughter said to me after the lecture, "You see mother how you are wasting your money on health foods".

Well, that did it. I told them flatly that I was going to continue to eat health foods, and if they wanted to swallow what that physical wreck told them, I would serve them what they wanted. I was boiling mad as I have tried to serve my family good, nutritious, nourishing foods from the health food store. For over five years only organically grown foods have been served at my table. From now on I will eat the health foods and I will serve my family just what they want, "junk". I will serve them canned fruit and vegetable juices while I will make my own juices from organically grown foods. I will make them mashed potatoes from the boxes filled with chemicals, as well as cake mixes, pancakes, processed cheese, T.V. frozen dinners, and all the dead-foods they desire.

How nutritionists can mix people up!

ANSWER:
You are so right . . . if your family wants poison, give it to them. The markets are full of it. Self-preservation is the first law of life, so you continue to go to your health food store and purchase your organically grown foods, your fertile eggs and all the other marvelous foods health stores have to offer. It's the best possible health insurance you can buy. I would rather you spend

your money on health foods than spend it with doctors, hospitals and drugs. You and I will bury all the dead-food eaters.

It is to be hoped that, in due course, your husband and daughter will discover for themselves the ill effects of "junk" foods . . . and return to your healthful way of eating.

QUESTION:

I am a very confused mother. At the cafeteria of the school where my children attend, the lunches are supervised by trained dieticians. Each week in our local paper the lunches for the coming week are published. They are supposed to be balanced, healthful meals for growing children. Meals including protein, starch, sugars, etc.

I herewith enclose a copy of a week's menus. Just look at the awful mess of "garbage" they are feeding the children — white bread exclusively, mashed and french fried potatoes, potato chips, pancakes, pork sausage, pizza pie, hot dogs, luncheon meats, fried chicken, white rice, greasy gravy, spaghetti, pickles, heavily sugared canned fruit, greasy oversalted soup, hydrogenated peanut butter and white sugar jelly, white bread, sandwiches, french toast with heavily sugared commerical syrup, chili, cakes, cookies, ice cream, and commercial puddings. Once in a while some pale lettuce, but fresh fruit never appears on any menu. Never whole wheat bread of honey.

I have been combatting this school lunch evil by preparing the lunches for my three children. I have been a health student of yours for years, and I firmly believe and follow a good nutritional program for my family.

But two of my children today refused to take their health lunches to school, claiming the other children tease them about their "funny food". Even their teacher told the children that the food at the cafeteria was well-balanced, nutritional food.

What is my next move? I am bewildered.

ANSWER:

When my five children attended school I was faced with the same evil situation. Just remember, the powerful food interests thoroughly control the food that is sold in all school cafeterias. They are special interest and have unlimited capital behind them. Don't expect any changes for the better in school cafeterias.

But you must do as I did. Go down to that school and tell the principal firmly that your children are not to enter the school cafeteria, then go to that ignorant school teacher and tell her she is to make no more sneering remarks about your children's lunches.

Then sit down with your three children and communicate with them. Give them home lessons in natural nutrition. Remember, life is a battle of capturing people's minds. Tell your children that the great food interests are trying to brainwash them into believing that the school food is nutritious food. Arouse their fighting instincts. Read them my books, have the natural health magazines like **Let's Live** available to them. Discuss this way of natural living with them. Don't let the great interests capture your children's minds. Tell your children there is vast difference between a school dietician and a dietician teaching natural nutrition. Explain the difference. Tell your children their teeth will decay, and they will become sick if they eat the cafeteria food.

QUESTION:

My mother has been placed in a convalescent rest home for old people. The food at this home is supervised by a hospital dietician. But you would never believe me when I tell you the "slop" they feed those poor old people. For breakfast they get gooey, mushy, cooked cereal covered with white sugar, pork sausage, hot cakes, bread and white sugar, jam and coffee. At lunch mashed potatoes and heavy greasy gravy, overcooked greasy meat, white rice, over-cooked frozen or canned vegetables and soft sponge cake and more coffee or tea. Dinner is usually a sloppy beef or lamb stew of some kind with grease floating on top, spaghetti, overboiled potatoes, sugary canned peas, white bread with margarine and some kind of white sugar dessert, ice cream or gelatin. Salads hardly ever

---

If mankind would at once discard all refined, sprayed, and unnatural foods, it would be the beginning of a race of people that would live long happy lives and be free of disease.
— Paul C. Bragg

Wisdom is the highest product of the human mind.
— Paul C. Bragg

appear on their trays, very little fruit. Sometimes they get a glass of commercial canned juice.

My mother is so constipated she is given an enema every day. She is pale, weak, and has lost the desire to live.

I have a big family and a small home and it is impossible to bring mother to my home. I am an only child. I want to help mother, but what can I do in a situation like this? My back is against a wall. I do not know what to do.

ANSWER:

This is a most difficult question for me to answer. I get hundreds of such letters from people like yourself who are forced to put their loved ones into a rest home for the aged.

I would suggest you give your mother natural food supplements from the health food store, and on every visit take fruits to her — apples, oranges, bananas and grapes. Make a finely cut salad, a bottle of carrot, beet and celery juice. A jar of freshly made salt-free vegetable soup. Take her dates, raisins, and apricots, and tell your mother to just soak the apricots in water overnight and eat them for breakfast. The Health Food Store has soft natural prunes she could eat. I would take her ground sunflower and sesame seeds.

It requires very little natural food to keep the human body healthy. And you can go to your health food store and tell them your problem and they will have many suggestions to improve your mother's nutrition. Where there is a will, there is a way. Don't let the dieticians kill your mother with their dead, devitalized foods.

The best service a book can render is to impart truth, but to make you think it out for yourself.
— **Elbert Hubbard**

Come forth into the light of things, let nature be your teacher.
— **Wordsworth**

It is time to dust off your dreams and shine up your ideas.
— **Paul C. Bragg**

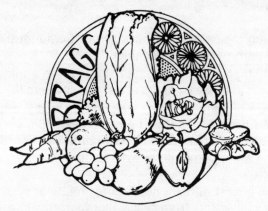

FROM THE AUTHORS

This book was written for YOU. It can be your passport to the Good Life. We Professional Nutritionists join hands in one common objective — a high standard of health for all and many added years to your life. Scientific Nutrition points the way — Nature's Way — the only lasting way to build a body free of degenerative diseases and premature aging. This book teaches you how to work with Nature and not against her. Doctors, dentists, and others who care for the sick, try to repair depleted tissues which too often mend poorly if at all. Many of them praise the spreading of this new scientific message of natural foods and methods for long-lasting health and youthfulness at any age. To speed the spreading of this tremendous message, this book was written.

Statements in this book are recitals of scientific findings, known facts of physiology, biological therapeutics, and reference to ancient writings as they are found. Paul C. Bragg has been practicing the natural methods of living for over 70 years, with highly beneficial results, knowing they are safe and of great value to others, and his daughter Patricia Bragg works with him to carry on the Health Crusade. They make no claims as to what the methods cited in this book will do for one in any given situation, and assume no obligation because of opinions expressed.

No cure for disease is offered in this book. No foods or diets are offered for the treatment or cure of any specific ailment. Nor is it intended as, or to be used as, literature for any food product. Paul C. Bragg and Patricia Bragg express their opinions solely as Public Health Educators, Professional Nutritionists and Teachers.

Certain persons considered experts may disagree with one or more statements in this book, as the same relate to various nutritional recommendations. However, any such statements are considered, nevertheless, to be factual, as based upon long-time experience of Paul C. Bragg and Patricia Bragg in the field of human health.

Please send Free Health Bulletins to these friends and relatives:

Name

Address

City   State   Zip Code

Name

Address

City   State   Zip Code

Name

Address

City   State   Zip Code

Name

Address

City   State   Zip Code

Name

Address

City   State   Zip Code

PLEASE SEND NAMES TO:

HEALTH SCIENCE, Box 310, Burbank, California 91503, U.S.A.

PLEASE CUT ALONG DOTTED LINE

Please send Free Health Bulletins to these friends and relatives:

Name

Address

City   State   Zip Code

. . . .

Name

Address

City   State   Zip Code

. . . .

Name

Address

City   State   Zip Code

. . . .

Name

Address

City   State   Zip Code

. . . .

Name

Address

City   State   Zip Code

. . . .

Name

Address

City   State   Zip Code

PLEASE CUT ALONG DOTTED LINE